An Aid to Diagnosis in Surg

To Professor Roy

In recognition of the high standards you set in Oman.

David Sellu. 13/6/95

An Aid to Diagnosis in Surgery

A practical manual for medical students

David Sellu, ChM, FRCS (Eng & Ed)
Consultant Surgeon and Senior Lecturer in Surgery
Ealing Hospital, Southall, Middlesex and
Hammersmith Hospital and Royal Postgraduate Medical School, London

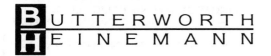

Butterworth-Heinemann Ltd
Linacre House, Jordan Hill, Oxford OX2 8DP

$\mathcal{R}$ A member of the Reed Elsevier plc group

OXFORD LONDON BOSTON
MUNICH NEW DELHI SINGAPORE SYDNEY
TOKYO TORONTO WELLINGTON

First published 1995

© Butterworth-Heinemann Ltd 1995

British Library Cataloguing in Publication Data
Sellu, David
    Aid to diagnosis in surgery: a practical
    manual for medical students
    I. Title
    617.075

Library of Congress Cataloguing in Publication Data
Sellu, David
    An aid to diagnosis in surgery: a practical manual for
    medical students/David Sellu
    p.   cm.
    Includes bibliographical references and index.
    1. Diagnosis, Surgical – Handbooks, manuals, etc.
    I. Title.
    [DNLM: 1. Diagnosis – handbooks.   WB 39 S468a]
    RD35.S44 1995
    616.07′54–dc20
    DNLM/DLC
    for Library of Congress   94–49105
                                                        CIP

ISBN 0 7506 2345 4

Printed and bound in Great Britain by
Biddles Ltd, Guildford and King's Lynn

Contents

Preface

The traditional method of history and examination, described in this book, continues to be taught in medical schools and hospitals throughout the world, despite calls to modify it. Although rigid, it has the merit of enabling the collection of comprehensive clinical information. This information is not simply to diagnose the presenting illness, although this is the prime objective. Among other things, it enables the student to learn to uncover intercurrent illness, potential drug interactions, and social and psychological problems.

Every medical student knows the frustration of trying to make a diagnosis from the large amount of information gained from this scheme. How should it be adapted to the presenting complaint? Which questions, out of the vast number memorized, will help in the given complaint? What do the symptoms obtained and signs elicited mean? This handbook provides some answers using a unique style based on this traditional approach, and provides a practical framework for a meaningful and rapid analysis of the history and examination.

* It is compact and can be carried easily in a white coat pocket.
* Its approach is problem orientated; it covers common symptoms, with a chapter devoted to each.
* For each symptom there is a classification of the causes and a handful of common and important causes.
* For each pathological condition there is a brief description of major symptoms and signs.
* Most of the remainder of the chapter is laid out in three columns indicating, for history, the reason for asking the questions that follow, the questions to ask the patient and the interpretation of the possible answers.
* For examination, you are told the reason for eliciting the signs that follow, a list of the signs and their relevance.

* The symptoms and signs that help most in reaching a diagnosis are highlighted for each complaint.
* In life-threatening conditions, resuscitation, history and examination are integrated to ensure prompt and effective management.
* The investigations required to confirm each of the more common conditions are discussed. I emphasize that the number of tests used for each problem is kept to a minimum.
* Sample case presentations illustrate each chapter. These are real patients treated either by me or one of my colleagues in a district hospital, the types of patients students are likely to encounter during their clerkships. The names given are fictitious. For more examples, I suggest the successful 'Case Presentations' series by Butterworths, which this book complements.

This layout encourages continuous analysis of the history and examination, enabling a sensible working diagnosis and rational use of radiological and laboratory tests. Only a selection of symptoms is covered, but the principles adopted can be applied to other clinical problems.

Inevitably, a book of this type lacks the details found in larger books. For example, it does not teach the student how to elicit signs in most instances, merely their interpretation. More detail will distract the student from the essential problem-solving process. In the column dealing with comments on the history and examination, I have had to make didactic statements for brevity. As each presenting problem is covered fairly comprehensively, there is repetition between chapters. This reduces the number of cross references. As an example, Chapter 2 deals with non-acute abdominal pain, while Chapter 3 describes the diagnosis of acute abdominal pain. Many of the questions asked and the signs elicited are similar but the subjects are sufficiently different to merit separate chapters.

I make no apologies for presenting the questions in the second column colloquially. A patient is more likely to understand 'pain in the navel area or around the belly button' than 'periumbilical pain'.

This book is intended as a pocket reference for junior surgical students not only during their clerkship but also when preparing for clinical examinations. I hope that senior students and house officers will find it beneficial. It presents an entirely new way of acquiring and interpreting conventional clinical data, a method I have taught successfully to medical students and junior doctors in the United Kingdom, Oman, in the Middle East and in Africa for the last 15 years.

Patients, students and doctors are referred to in the male gender simply to avoid awkward expressions such as 'he or she', 'him or her' and 'himself or herself'. I apologize for this.

David Sellu
Department of Surgery
Hammersmith Hospital and Royal Postgraduate Medical School
London

Acknowledgements

Conscious of the novel nature of this book and the readership for whom it is intended, I sought help from several experts, all active teachers of undergraduate medical students. There are too many to acknowledge here, but I am particularly grateful to my colleagues Pierce Grace, Eamonn Kiely, Susan Carter and Simon Choong, and to Professors Harold Ellis and Tim de Dombal for patiently going through the manuscript and making valuable suggestions. Pierce has agreed to collaborate with me to produce an electronic version of this book.

I am particularly grateful to the medical students in Oman, to whom I taught this method of clinical data analysis. They helped me refine many of the questions and proved that this technique works well.

Geoff Smaldon and his staff at Butterworth-Heinemann have given the usual high standard of technical support, for which I am most grateful. Finally, my thanks go once again to my wife Catherine and our children Amy, Daniel, Sophie and James for their help and encouragement. They know most of the questions in this book and the answers by heart.

Introduction

Abbreviations used in this book

During history and examination

PC	Presenting complaint(s)
HPC	History of presenting complaints
ROS	Review of systems
GIS or GIT	Gastrointestinal system or tract
RS	Respiratory system
GUS	Genito-urinary system
CVS	Cardiovascular system
CNS	(Central) nervous system
PMH	Past medical history
FH	Family history
SH	Social history
JVP	Jugular venous pressure

Investigations

Hb	Haemoglobin
FBC	Full blood count
WCC	White cell count
PCV	Packed cell volume (haematocrit)
ESR	Erythrocyte sedimentation rate
CRP	C reactive protein
U&Es	Urea and electrolytes
LFTs	Liver function tests
TFTs	Thyroid function tests
ECG	Electrocardiogram
CT	Computerized tomography
MRI	Magnetic resonance imaging
ERCP	Endoscopic retrograde cholangio-pancreatography

Treatment

NSAID	Non-steroidal anti-inflammatory drug
IV	Intravenous

Diseases

TB	Tuberculosis
Ca	Carcinoma

Structure of this book

Broadly speaking, as a student you will participate in the management of two types of patients: those who can be investigated without dire urgency, and those with life-threatening or potentially fatal conditions. An example of the former is a patient with varicose veins and of the latter, one with upper gastrointestinal bleeding. In the latter case, resuscitation takes priority after preliminary assessment; full history is taken and physical examination completed as soon as the patient's condition permits.

This book is laid out as follows:

Symptom

Introduction/definition/significance of symptom

Classification of causes

This is usually an anatomical or physiological classi-fication that ensures important causes are not over-looked.

Common and important causes

A short list is given of common or important causes of the symptom. While you must concentrate on the recognition of common disorders, you must not ignore rare, though important, diseases, or those easy to recognize from clinical features. For example, car-cinoma of the thyroid is an uncommon but important cause of dysphagia, and it is easy to feel for lumps in the thyroid. You must always examine the thyroid in a patient with dysphagia.

The percentages given here and elsewhere in this book indicate the relative frequency of disorders, symptoms or signs discussed. These figures have been obtained mainly from publications over the last few years on workload from district general hospitals.

Points to look for

This is a synopsis of the clinical features of each common condition. It is given at this stage to focus your mind on the characteristics that will help you make a diagnosis.

History

This is under the following headings:

(a) Reason for interrogation
(b) Questions asked
(c) Comments

The questions you ask the patient are often printed but, in some places, only an indication is given of what to ask. There are good and bad ways of asking questions during history taking. Some of the questions given, even though in colloquial language, will need to be modified so as not to mislead. They are presented this way for brevity. De Dombal (1993) has given an excellent account of how to interview patients to get unbiased answers, and I recommend his book.

The crucial opening question in history taking is one that allows the patient to tell the history in his own words, for example, 'Please can you tell me what the matter is, from the beginning?' or 'Please can you tell me all the things that you have noticed wrong?' To avoid repetition, this question is omitted throughout, but is important.

In a few places, Questions asked and Comments (and Signs elicited and Comments) are combined to make for easier reading.

Examination

This is under the following headings:

(a) Reason for examination
(b) Signs looked for
(c) Comments

The features in the history and examination that help most in diagnosis and management are highlighted by italics. If the highlight is in the left hand columns, all items against it to the right must be taken to be important.

Investigations

The investigations required to make a diagnosis of each major condition are listed and discussed.

Making a clinical diagnosis

There are several ways of making a diagnosis. The most common is by pattern recognition. You start by learning the common symptoms and signs of diseases and note variations in clinical presentation. When you encounter a patient in whom you wish to make a diagnosis, you take a history and perform an examination. You compare your findings with the features of known disorders until you discover a reasonable match. In classic cases, the match may be almost perfect; in most instances, however, some features may not fit well, but a pattern can still be recognized. Appreciating these variations in the presentation of a given condition takes time and experience but a systematic and analytical approach, as presented in this book, will help you make a list of probable diagnoses. Remember, however, that no method of clinical data interpretation gives the correct diagnosis every time.

Case report

At the end of each chapter is an illustrative presentation together with detailed analyses. Try and do your own evaluation of the features presented and see how your answers compare with mine. As a student, avoid obscure conditions and remember that common things are common. When you finish reading a chapter, try the corresponding case in the 'Case Presentations' series.

References

References are listed at the end of some chapters.

Clinical history and examination

The following method of history and examination is taught and used most frequently in hospitals throughout the United Kingdom and other countries. It encourages you as a junior student to take a complete history and do a full examination. With more experience, you will be able to omit certain questions and parts of the examination and still make a good working diagnosis. Some of the symptoms and signs below are defined and their significance indicated. Avoid making your diagnosis from a single symptom or sign and keep an open mind until you have analysed all the evidence gained from history and examination. Adopt what de Dombal calls a 'probabilistic' approach (de Dombal, 1991): most students will make a diagnosis of appendicitis only if there is pain in the right lower quadrant of the abdomen. Yet, as many as 25% of patients with this diagnosis do not have pain in the right lower quadrant. Right lower quadrant pain makes the diagnosis of appendicitis more likely, but its absence does not exclude it.

The classic features of disease presented in this and other books are not always present, especially in the early stages, or may be modified by a number of external factors such as medications. Remember also the complex interaction between body and mind and the way it affects the presentation of a given disease from one individual to another. For example, anaemia may present with chest pain in one patient, breathlessness in another, and in others lethargy. Physical symptoms may be due to psychogenic causes and psychiatric symptoms may be the first manifestation of organic disease. Weight loss, for example, may be due to depression or to diabetes mellitus; and depression may be the earliest feature of malignancy or use of illicit drugs.

All the terms used in this chapter are defined in Browse's *An Introduction to the Symptoms and Signs of Surgical Disease*. They are presented here for ready reference. Some are described. During history and examination, refer to this chapter to be sure you do not miss major symptoms or signs.

Introductions

Introduce yourself first, making clear to the patient that you are a junior student, and ask him to introduce himself (Browse, 1993; Hope *et al.*, 1989). Note his full name, age, sex, occupation and marital status. Give a brief description of his home now and details later in the social history.

History

Presenting complaints

List all the presenting complaints in chronological order. Avoid leading questions and let the patient tell his own story. Encourage the patient with 'Is there anything else wrong?' or 'Are there any other problems I ought to know about?' When making a note of your findings, rewrite all colloquial expressions in proper 'medical' English except where a direct quotation of the patient's own words conveys the meaning better.

Example:

Intermittent dull pain in the epigastrium for 12 months
Jaundice for 4 weeks

History of presenting complaints

Describe the symptoms listed in the presenting complaints. Again, listen to what the patient has to say.
For *pain* ask about:

When first noticed
Location
Radiation
Mode of onset (sudden or gradual)
Quality or description of pain (Browse, 1993)
How it has progressed since onset (getting better or worse?)
Continuous or intermittent
If continuous, how it is progressing
If intermittent, duration, length of intervals of freedom, frequency
Aggravating and relieving factors

Relation to events such as the time of day, food, coughing, micturition, defecation, movement, posture

Associated features such as vomiting, visual disturbance (e.g. migraine), fever etc.

Any special qualities of pain

For *lump* ask about:

Whether single or multiple
Location(s)
How long it has been present
Whether getting bigger, smaller, constant or varying
Whether painful or painless
Discharge from lump or vicinity; if so describe
Any associated features, e.g. relation to periods in the case of breast lump
Further enquiries into the system to which the presenting symptoms belong

Review of systems

Gastrointestinal system (start from above down)

Appetite
Weight changes: weight loss is an important symptom. Attempt to establish amount of weight lost by asking the following questions:

What is your normal weight?
When was your weight last normal?
What is your weight now?
How well do your clothes fit?
Those who weigh themselves regularly will be able to tell you how much weight they have lost. Those who do not will realize they have lost weight because their clothes are getting loose.

Teeth, natural or prosthetic
Soreness of mouth, throat, gums; dryness of mouth, thirst
Pain and swelling of salivary glands
Regurgitation: this is the expulsion of food without effort
Nausea, vomiting, haematemesis

Dysphagia: this is difficulty in swallowing.

Waterbrash: this is excessive secretion of saliva. When associated with heartburn it is believed to be a protective response to gastro-esophageal reflux. The excess saliva helps to neutralize acid in the oesophagus (Helm, 1986).

Heartburn (epigastric or retrosternal burning sensation spreading up to the throat)

Abdominal pain (describe as above under pain)

Epigastric/retrosternal pain or discomfort usually related to meals. Many of these patients have no abnormality on endoscopy.

When an abnormality is found, it is most likely to be oesophagitis, duodenal ulcer or duodenitis, hiatus hernia or gastric ulcer. Gastric cancer is an uncommon cause but one that should be suspected if a middle-aged or elderly patient complains of epigastric pain of recent onset (6 months or less).

Flatulence: this is excessive wind. It may be in the form of belching, abdominal distension or passage of flatus per rectum.

Excessive belching is usually not due to organic disease and is a common functional symptom. It is due to excessive air swallowing.

Jaundice, colour of stools and urine: jaundice is defined as a yellow discoloration of the skin and mucous membranes due to staining with bilirubin when the plasma concentration is more than 18 μmol/l but clinically detectable only at higher concentrations. Pale or putty coloured stools and dark urine suggest intra- or extrahepatic biliary obstruction; pruritus may be present.

Abdominal distension: distension must be distinguished from obesity.

Abdominal mass: some patients present with a lump in the abdomen.

Bowel habits, diarrhoea, constipation: establish the patient's normal bowel pattern by noting the frequency of bowel movement, the consistency and description (colour, amount) of the stools; and whether there has been any recent change in this pattern.

Use of aperients: determine whether the patient uses any opening medicines, and if so the name, dose, frequency and duration of any medication used. Laxative abuse is a common and under-recognized cause of diarrhoea. Other features include abdominal pain, weight loss, nausea and hypokalaemia. It is commoner in female patients.

Bleeding per rectum: amount and colour of blood; mixed with stools or on toilet paper, or in the toilet bowl?

Mucus, other discharge from anus. Mucus is passed per rectum in inflammatory bowel disease, from tumours and bowel infections.

Ano-rectal

Pain
Pruritus (itching)
Lumps at anal verge, whether they prolapse; ability to reduce spontaneously or manually. Haemorrhoids are the most common lumps that prolapse at the anal verge. Classification of haemorrhoids into first, second and third degree depends on whether they prolapse and reduce. First degree haemorrhoids do not prolapse; second degree haemorrhoids prolapse and reduce spontaneously or can be pushed back. Third degree haemorrhoids are out all the time and cannot be pushed back.

Polyps in the rectum can also prolapse during defecation.
Tenesmus: a sensation felt in the rectum of incomplete evacuation after defecation. It is as if there is something still there that cannot be passed. It is common in the irritable bowel syndrome and may be caused by a rectal tumour.

Bowel habit (as above)

Respiratory system

Cough
Dyspnoea
Stridor, wheezing
Haemoptysis

Pleuritic chest pain
Occupational exposure, pets, allergens
Night sweats and weight loss (possibility of
  tuberculosis or lymphoma)
Origin from Indian subcontinent, Africa or Far
  East (for instance when TB is suspected)

Genito-urinary system

Genital system

Marital status
If married, for how long?
Sexual activities (e.g. suspected sexually
  transmitted disease)
Sexual orientation (heterosexual, homosexual or
  bisexual)
History of venereal infection
Difficulties with ejaculation or orgasm
Difficulties with fertility

Males

Urethral discharge (describe)

Penile lesions
Difficulties with sexual intercourse

Females (include obstetric history)

Age at menarche
Pregnancies
Deliveries/live births/still births; did she breast
  feed? If yes, how long for each child?
Dyspareunia (pain on sexual intercourse)
Post-coital bleeding
Periods
  Regular or irregular
  For how many days does she bleed?
  How long between periods (i.e. from day 1 of
    one to day 1 of the next)?
  Loss, any clots
  Pain
  Other symptoms e.g. depression, irritability
  Intermenstrual bleeding
Vaginal discharge (describe)
Vulval lesions
Age at menopause, if appropriate
  Post-menopausal bleeding

Urinary system

Thirst, fluid intake
Polyuria
Symptoms of chronic renal failure: in severe renal failure, nearly every system is affected (Kumar and Clark, 1994). These include anaemia (lethargy, breathlessness), the central nervous system (confusion, coma and fits in severe cases), the kidneys (polyuria, oedema), gastrointestinal system (anorexia, nausea, diarrhoea).
Loin pain
Fever, rigors
Frequency of micturition, nocturia
Pain on micturition
Urgency of micturition
Hesitancy before micturition
Force of urinary stream
Dribbling
Length of time it takes to empty bladder
Incontinence, and if present, precipitating factors, for example coughing, straining
History of acute retention of urine

Haematuria
Debris or gravel in the urine
Passage of urinary tract stones

Breast symptoms

Lump(s)
Pain, discomfort in breast
Discharge
Ulcer or rash on breast

Cardiovascular system

Chest pain, angina
Palpitations
Dyspnoea
Orthopnoea (breathlessness on lying flat): it is caused by pulmonary congestion in the flat position, and is due to left ventricular failure. It improves when the patient assumes the upright position.

Paroxysmal nocturnal dyspnoea (breathlessness which wakes the patient up from sleep). The mechanisms are similar to orthopnoea. The failing left ventricle is unable to match the output of the more normal right ventricle, and this results in pulmonary oedema. It may also be a symptom of bronchial asthma.

Syncope: sudden transient loss of consciousness. There are many causes of syncope, and not all are due to cardiac disease. Cardiac causes include third degree atrioventricular block, aortic stenosis and paroxysmal supraventricular tachycardia. Some non-cardiac causes are cerebrovascular disease and drugs such as nitroglycerine.

Ankle oedema
Intermittent claudication (Chapter 15)
Varicose veins
Ulceration of the leg
Recent dental treatment (suspicion of bacterial endocarditis)
History of rheumatic fever

Nervous system

Handedness (right or left)
Difficulty with walking, type of gait
Headaches
Unconsciousness
Dizziness, fainting attacks, blackouts
Fits, epilepsy
Visual disturbance: does the patient wear glasses?
Hearing problems, hearing aids
Disturbance of sense of smell and taste
Muscle weakness
Sensory impairment
Disturbance of behaviour, mood, personality; hallucinations; drive

Musculo-skeletal system

Pain in muscles, joints and bones
Swelling and stiffness of joints and relation to rest, exercise, etc; and time of day, e.g. early morning stiffness
Difficulty with walking/abnormal gait

Past medical history

Past illnesses and operations and their dates
Injuries and accidents and dates
Enquire about specific diseases:

  Diabetes
  Hypertension
  Renal disease
  Heart disease
  Respiratory illness such as bronchitis, asthma
    and TB
  Epilepsy
  Jaundice
  Stroke

In women, past obstetric history, if not obtained
above in genital system

Family history

Draw a family tree of immediate relatives and
note serious illnesses and causes of death when
hereditary diseases are suspected.

Drugs

*Note dose, frequency, route of administration and
  duration of each important drug*
Insulin and other antidiabetic agents
Steroids currently taken or taken in the past;
  NSAIDs
Antihypertensive drugs
Oral contraceptive pill
Anticoagulants
Anticonvulsants
All current medications

Allergies

Allergens and the response the patient has when
exposed

Social history

House and home conditions
Marital status, children; previous marriages and
  any spouses and children being supported

Occupation including job actually performed, wages, satisfaction with job

Leisure and hobbies

Racial, ethnic, religious and cultural background (McKenzie and Crowcroft, 1994)

Recent life crises such as illness or bereavement

Major events in the family such as pregnancy

Habits such as smoking and drinking (number of cigarettes smoked per day or ounces of tobacco per week; number of units of alcohol consumed per week.

Use of illicit drugs

Examination

General examination

Race and ethnic background
General condition
Physiological age
Ill/well
Obese/cachectic
Appearance, cleanliness
Intellect, mood, memory, personality

Abnormal pigmentation
Posture, facies, obvious anomalies
Anaemia, pallor
Cyanosis
Jaundice
Rash
Body and scalp hair
Lymph nodes: occipital, preauricular, submandibular, cervical, supraclavicular, axillary, epitrochlear, inguinal areas
Thyroid gland
Skull, neck, spine, trunk, limbs: note signs of injury or operation
Tongue: dry, glossitis, ulcer
Clubbing of fingers/toes

Full examination of the breasts and axillae

If lump found anywhere, describe:

Site
Tissue plane in which lump lies (in dermis, subcutaneous, intramuscular, etc.)
What it is attached to

Size
Shape
Surface
Consistency
Mobility in relation to nearby structures
Colour
Tenderness
Temperature
Pulsation
Fluctuation
Bruit or thrill
Transillumination
Cough impulse where relevant
Associated lumps
Other features
Regional lymph node enlargement

If ulcer found, describe:

Site
Size
Shape
Painful or tender
State of surrounding tissues: swelling,
   temperature, etc.

Margin (e.g. rolled, raised and everted in some
   malignancies)
Other features
Regional lymph nodes

Cardiovascular system

Blood pressure, in both arms whenever possible
Pulse: rate, rhythm, volume, nature of the arterial
   wall
Jugular venous pressure
Apex beat
Palpable thrills

Cardiac size on percussion
Heart sounds, murmurs, rubs and other sounds
Vascular examination of the limbs including
   peripheral pulses. See Chapters 15 and 16

Respiratory system

Deformities of the chest wall
Respiratory rate, volume, pattern
Position of the trachea

Regional lymph nodes

Chest expansion

Tactile fremitus: increased in consolidation, diminished or absent in pleural effusion, pneumothorax and lung collapse.

Percussion note: the resonance is increased in emphysema, pneumothorax; decreased in lung collapse, consolidation; stony dull in pleural effusion, haemothorax and empyema of the thorax.

Air entry

Breath sounds: bronchial breath sounds are heard in consolidation of the lung; breath sounds are reduced if there is a pleural effusion, pneumothorax, or lung collapse.

Added sounds: wheezes, crackles, pleural rubs. Wheezes are heard in obstructive airways disease such as asthma or bronchitis. Low pitched crackles are present when the air passages are filled with mucus or pus. Fine crackles are present over areas of consolidation and pulmonary oedema.

Examination of the abdomen

Inspection

Scars, incisional hernias

Distension: if present, what is distending? Fluid, faeces, flatus, fetus, fibroid, fat, full bladder

Distended veins

Skin discoloration

Visible peristalsis

Pulsation

Masses

Palpation

Tenderness: if present, is there muscle guarding and rebound tenderness?

Systematic examination of the normal viscera

If mass found, what are its characteristics (see Introduction) and its relation to normal structures?

Is it in the abdominal wall, within the peritoneum or is it retroperitoneal?

Feel for thrills, which can occur over narrowed
   arteries
Examine regional lymph nodes

Percussion

Percuss over abdomen
Percuss for dullness over liver and spleen
Percuss over any masses found
Test for shifting dullness

Auscultation

Bowel sounds
Bruits
Succussion splash

Examination of the groins

Inspection

Swelling
Discoloration
Visible cough impulse

Palpation

Mass
Tenderness
Pulsation
Reducibility
Expansile cough impulse
Thrills
Regional lymph nodes

Auscultation

Bruits

Examination of the scrotum

Is the scrotal sac normal and well developed?
Are there two normal testes?
If a swelling is present:

   can you get above it?
   can you feel it separately from the testis?
   does the testis feel normal?
   is the epididymis normal?
   define the characteristics of the swelling.
   does it transilluminate?
   is it more prominent on standing or straining?
Is there tenderness? Exactly where?

Examination of the rectum (described in detail in Chapter 6)

Examination of the lower limb (described in Chapters 15 and 16)

Nervous system

General
Speech
Gait
Intellect
Cranial nerves (numbers correspond to the nerves):

1. Sense of smell
2. Examine fundi
   Visual acuity
   Visual fields
3, 4, 6. Inspect lids, pupils, direction of gaze of each eyeball
   Pupillary reflexes
   Ocular movements
   Any nystagmus?
5. Sensation on face
   Corneal reflexes
   Muscles of mastication
   Jaw jerk
7. Muscles of facial expression
   Taste anterior two-thirds of tongue
8. Test hearing
   Rinne's and Weber's tests
9. Sensation posterior two-thirds of tongue
10. Voice
    Movement of palate
11. Sternocleidomastoid and trapezius muscles: patient to shrug shoulders and to press chin against your hand
12. Tongue movement

Motor system

Involuntary movements
Abnormal postures
Wasting, fasciculations
Power
Tone, clonus
Coordination

Sensory system

Temperature
Touch
Superficial and deep pain
Position and vibration sense

Reflexes

Others

Neck stiffness

Investigations

When planning investigations, it is important first to consider whether a test is necessary at all. In many instances in surgery, diagnosis can be made without tests. If investigations are required, those which are cheap, easy to perform and do not inflict pain on, or cause inconvenience to, the patient, must be done before the difficult, expensive and invasive ones. In many more cases the answers will be obtained with few investigations. One way to observe this principle is to think of tests in the following rough order. This is by no means an absolute order, but is given merely as a guide. In a patient with clinical features suggesting acute cholecystitis, ultrasound of the upper abdomen is performed early and oral cholecystogram, if at all indicated, will be done much later when the symptoms have subsided. In some cases the diagnosis is obtained by one or two tests; all others are omitted. For example, in a patient with dysphagia due to carcinoma of the oesophagus, a barium swallow will show a typical filling defect in the oesophagus and upper gastrointestinal endoscopy allows visualization and biopsy of the lesion. Chest X-ray and ultrasound of the abdomen are done to determine whether secondaries are present.

Some of the indications for these tests are discussed below.

(a) *Urine tests:* appearance of urine, ward tests (urinalysis for protein, blood, sugar, bilirubin, urobilinogen, pH, specific gravity). Ward testing of urine is a useful screen for every patient as it picks up many cases of undiagnosed disease such as diabetes mellitus. Laboratory tests (e.g. culture and sensitivity, urinary cytology when carcinoma is suspected in the urinary tract, urinary biochemistry). Useful in suspected urinary tract disorders such as stone, infection and tumour; in the investigation of jaundice.

(b) *Stool tests:* ward observations (frequency of stools, the colour, volume and consistency and odour; presence of blood or mucus); laboratory tests (testing for blood, looking for ova and parasites, culture). Useful in patients with inflammatory bowel disease, stool infection and when malignancy suspected. The stool is pale or putty coloured in obstructive jaundice.

(c) *Microbiological tests:* sputum culture, blood culture, wound swabs, throat and vaginal swabs, etc. Useful when investigating infections of the respiratory tract and wounds; in suspected septicaemia.

(d) *Blood tests:*

   (i) *Haematological tests:* Hb, FBC, ESR or CRP, clotting screening. Hb and FBC used widely to confirm or refute the presence of anaemia, for instance in chronic bleeding or suspected malignancy; ESR and CRP are not specific but gross elevation should alert you to the presence of infection, inflammatory disorder or malignancy. Clotting screening is useful in suspected clotting disorders such as in obstructive jaundice.

   (ii) *Blood U&Es, LFTs, glucose, TFTs, amylase, other biochemical tests:* U&Es carried out in patients who present with excessive fluid loss such as in vomiting or diarrhoea; or in renal disorders. LFTs are useful in liver disease, in suspected or confirmed metastatic cancer to the liver. Calcium and plasma proteins are often measured as part of LFTs and are useful in patients with suspected derangements of calcium metabolism (for instance hyperparathyroidism); plasma proteins are useful in assessing nutritional status.

   Blood glucose is measured when diabetes or hypoglycaemia suspected; also to monitor the treatment of diabetes. TFTs are performed when investigating thyroid disorder such as hyper- or hypothyroidism, and some instances of goitre. Amylase is measured if acute pancreatitis suspected.

(e) *ECG:* cardiac disease is important for the surgeon in many ways particularly if surgery is contemplated. Cardiac disorders sometimes aggravate surgical disease, for instance, intermittent claudication is made worse by cardiac failure owing to reduced oxygen supply to the limbs. Cardiac disease may produce surgical symptoms, for example dysphagia due to pressure on and obstruction of the oesophagus from cardiac enlargement; or emboli to the limb arteries from a thrombus in the left atrium. Intercurrent cardiac disease is one of the commonest causes of morbidity and death following operations. ECG can show cardiac rate and rhythm, myocardial ischaemia, ventricular hypertrophy and other disorders of cardiac morphology and function.

(f) *X-rays:*

   (i) *Plain X-rays* must always be considered before those in which contrast such as barium is given.

   (ii) *Contrast X-rays:* e.g. barium meal, IVU, oral cholecystogram.

(g) *Special imaging techniques:*

   (i) *Ultrasound scanning:* this procedure is especially useful because it is non-invasive and can be done with little preparation of the patient. It is used widely in the investigation of disorders of the liver (e.g. malignancy), biliary tract (e.g. stone disease), pancreas (e.g. tumour), kidneys and urinary tract (e.g. tumours and obstruction) and other intra- and extraperitoneal disorders.

   (ii) *Isotope scanning*, e.g. of the liver and bones. Isotopes are useful in detecting abnormalities such as tumours in the liver. Bone scans used in investigating suspected secondary deposits in bone from primary tumours elsewhere, for example the thyroid.

Technetium and iodine scans are used in investigating thyroid dysfunction and goitre.

(iii) *CT scanning:* this procedure gives images of very high quality, but is expensive and is not available in all hospitals. Its most common use is in investigating suspected intra-abdominal malignancy but is useful for imaging disease at other sites, for instance hard and soft tissue malignancies in the limbs.

(iv) *Magnetic resonance scanning* is superior to CT scanning in some instances, but is even more expensive and less widely available.

(h) *Endoscopic investigations:* all endoscopic investigations allow visualization of the tract for which they are designed; suspicious lesions can be biopsied. They all provide facilities for therapy, for instance excision of certain benign tumours and extraction of foreign bodies. Benign strictures can be dilated or widened in other ways.

(i) *Upper gastro-intestinal tract endoscopy:* for viewing the oropharynx, oesophagus, stomach and duodenum. It is useful for injecting oesophageal varices and extracting foreign bodies. Benign strictures can be dilated and malignant ones intubated during this procedure.

(ii) *Sigmoidoscopy:* used in inspection of the rectum and lower sigmoid colon. As in other endoscopic examinations, biopsies can be taken and certain lesions treated; through the sigmoidoscope, polyps can be excised and foreign bodies extracted.

(iii) *Bronchoscopy:* allows examination of the bronchial tree.

(iv) *Urethro-cystoscopy:* for the inspection of the urinary tract. A ureteroscope can be passed to examine the ureters and renal pelvis.

(v) *ERCP:* in this examination, a fibreoptic endoscope is passed through the mouth, oesophagus and stomach to the duodenum. The upper gastrointestinal tract is carefully inspected first. The duodenal papilla is identified and cannulated and contrast injected through it to outline the biliary and pancreatic ducts. It can show tumours, benign strictures, stones and other diseases of these organs. The sphincter of Oddi, if narrowed, can be divided to allow more free drainage of the biliary and pancreatic systems. A stent can be inserted into the lower end of the common bile duct to treat a stricture.

(vi) *Colonoscopy:* in expert hands the whole of the colon can be inspected. Suspicious lesions can be biopsied and polyps excised.

(vii) *Laparoscopy:* this procedure is used widely in diagnosing intraperitoneal diseases such as those affecting the liver, lymph nodes, stomach, appendix and pelvic organs. A wide variety of operations is now possible with the aid of laparoscopy, for instance cholecystectomy, repair of hiatus and groin hernias, appendicectomy and colectomy.

(i) *Operative investigations:* these include biopsy of suspicious lesions of skin, lymph node, liver, breast and other organs.

(j) *Laparotomy:* this is now used rarely as a diagnostic procedure because of the availability of specialized scans and laparoscopy.

In the synopsis that follows, only the symptoms and signs relevant to the problem stated will be described in detail, but you must include all the other symptoms and signs to complete the clinical investigation.

References

Browse, N. (1993) *An Introduction to the Symptoms and Signs of Surgical Disease* (second edition). Edward Arnold, London.

de Dombal, F. T. (1991) *Diagnosis of Acute Abdominal Pain* (second edition). Churchill Livingstone, Edinburgh.

de Dombal, F. T. (1993) *Surgical Decision Making*. Butterworth-Heinemann, Oxford.

Helm, J. F. (1986) Esophageal acid clearance. *Journal of Clinical Gastroenterology*, **8** (supplement 1), 5–11.

Hope, R. A., Longmore, J. M., Hodgetts, T. J., Ramrakha, P. S. (1994) *Oxford Handbook of Clinical Medicine* (third edition). Oxford University Press, Oxford.

Kumar, P. J., Clark, M. L. (editors) (1994) *Clinical Medicine*. Baillière Tindall, London, p. 173.

McKenzie, K. J., Crowcroft, N. S. (1994) Race, ethnicity, culture and science. *British Medical Journal*, **6950**, 286–287.

Further reading

Browse, N. (1993) *An Introduction to the Symptoms and Signs of Surgical Disease* (second edition). Edward Arnold, London.

Clain, A. (editor) (1986) *Hamilton Bailey's Demonstration of Physical Signs in Clinical Surgery* (seventh edition). Wright, Bristol.

de Dombal, F. T. (1991) *Diagnosis of Acute Abdominal Pain* (second edition). Churchill Livingstone, Edinburgh.

Hobsley, M. (1991) *Pathways in Surgical Management* (second edition). Edward Arnold, London.

Titles in the 'Case Presentation' series by Butterworth-Heinemann:

Case Presentations in Arterial Disease
Case Presentations in Clinical Geriatric Medicine
Case Presentations in Endocrinology and Diabetes
Case Presentations in Gastrointestinal Disease
Case Presentations in General Surgery
Case Presentations in Heart Disease
Case Presentations in Medical Ophthalmology
Case Presentations in Neurology
Case Presentations in Obstetrics and Gynaecology
Case Presentations in Otolaryngology
Case Presentations in Paediatrics
Case Presentations in Renal Medicine
Case Presentations in Respiratory Medicine

Chapter 1

Dysphagia

Dysphagia is difficulty in swallowing. The difficulty may be due to local causes, neurological disorders or disturbance of motility, or to pain in the oropharynx. The patient complains of a sensation of food sticking and may localize it to anywhere between the hyoid bone and the epigastrium. The site pointed to does not correspond well with site of obstruction, and should be disregarded. Dysphagia is a distressing and dangerous symptom, which should be investigated fully unless there is an obvious cause such as oral or pharyngeal infection.

History is more important than examination in a patient presenting with dysphagia. It is rare to encounter patients with severe malnutrition or signs of disseminated malignancy. In most, there are few or no signs.

Causes of dysphagia

Anatomical classification

In the lumen	In the wall	Outside the wall	Neurological causes	Others
Foreign bodies	Carcinoma of the pharynx, oesophagus or stomach Benign stricture, e.g. due to peptic oesophagitis with or without hiatus hernia, or oesophagoscopy or corrosive injury Achalasia of oesophagus Congenital stricture	Pharyngeal pouch Carcinoma bronchus Cardiac enlargement Enlarged thyroid gland Lymphoma and mediastinal nodes	Bulbar palsy Myasthenia gravis	Globus hystericus

Clinical classification (Hobsley, 1989)

Acute	*Chronic*
Corrosive injury	Other causes listed above
Foreign body	
Acute inflammation of the mouth and pharynx	

Common causes	Benign stricture (40%), carcinoma of the oesophagus (30%), foreign bodies (5%), carcinoma of stomach (4%)
Rare but important causes	Achalasia of oesophagus ($<1\%$), carcinoma of the pharynx ($<1\%$), ingestion of corrosive substance ($<1\%$)
	Do not forget oesophageal atresia or tracheo-oesophageal fistula as a cause of dysphagia in neonates.

Points to look for

Benign oesophageal stricture

Patient middle-aged or elderly, often female.
History of waterbrash, heartburn and epigastric
  pain, suggesting pre-existing hiatus hernia.
Symptoms may remit and are often more slowly
  progressive than in a patient with carcinoma.
Dysphagia present for years rather than
  months.
The patient usually looks well and may be obese.

Carcinoma of oesophagus

85% occur in patients over 65 years of age and it
  is often painless.

2

Males more commonly affected (60%).

More common in those from southern Africa and China.

Dysphagia initially for solids but semi-solids and liquids affected later, and saliva if obstruction total.

Dysphagia present for weeks or a few months rather than years.

Coughing bouts in the night suggest spillage of oesophageal contents or saliva into the bronchial tree.

Anorexia, malaise and weight loss present in later stages.

Patient malnourished and anaemic in 15%.

Cervical lymph nodes, lung collapse or consolidation and hepatomegaly suggest secondaries.

Foreign bodies in oesophagus

Produce acute dysphagia (90%). In some, dysphagia does not occur.

Suspect in the very young or old with dysphagia.

There is often (90%) but not invariably a history of ingestion of foreign body.

Foreign body impaction commoner at the site of pre-existing abnormality such as benign stricture.

Carcinoma of stomach

Patient aged over 65 years in 85% of cases.

Anorexia, malaise and weight loss present in 55%.

Dyspepsia less than 6 months in 75%.

Anaemia (15%).

Dysphagia is a late presenting complaint of carcinoma of the stomach.

Dysphagia as a presenting feature of carcinoma of the stomach occurs in 4% of patients with this malignancy.

Achalasia of oesophagus

Most common in patients aged 20–40 years of age. 85% of achalasia occurs in this age group.

Dysphagia associated with pain on swallowing both fluids and solids occurs in 75% of those with achalasia.

Symptoms slowly progressive and may be present for many years.

80% of patients with achalasia present after experiencing symptoms for over 18 months.

75% of patients find it easier to swallow solids rather than liquids.

Malnutrition and aspiration pneumonia occur in less than 5% of those with achalasia.

History

Reason for questions	Questions asked	Comment
Find out about dysphagia, its onset, progression and severity	When could you last swallow normally? When did you first notice difficulty in swallowing? What could you swallow easily then? (see below)	
	How did the difficulty in swallowing start? Was it sudden or did it start gradually?	The speed with which dysphagia occurs depends on the cause: a malignant stricture often produces abrupt difficulty and progresses over weeks or months to total dysphagia. If the stricture is benign, dysphagia starts gradually and progresses slowly. In acute, total and painful dysphagia, suspect oropharyngeal infection

	Do you have difficulty swallowing every time you eat, or only sometimes?	Continuous in malignancy in over 90%; variable in achalasia in 85%
	What can and can you not swallow? Can you swallow solids (e.g. an apple)? Can you swallow semi-solids (e.g. porridge)? Can you swallow liquids (e.g. tea or water)? Can you swallow your own saliva?	75% of patients with achalasia find it easier to swallow solids than liquids Inability to swallow saliva means total obstruction
	Can you drink liquids quickly?	If he cannot, he may have a neurological cause or achalasia. Neurological lesions together account for less than 3% of the causes of dysphagia
	Do you bring your food or drink back up? (i.e. regurgitate)	Risk of aspiration pneumonia. Aspiration pneumonia occurs in less than 3% of all patients with dysphagia
Describe events during a typical meal. *They give clues to a possible cause.*	Let us assume you are given a plate of food now. Can you describe to me what happens from when you start eating to when you finish?	Allow the patient to describe in his own words the sequence of events which occur during a meal It may be necessary to ask direct questions to clarify certain points below:
Malignancy	What is your appetite like? (Does patient have anorexia?) How do you feel in yourself? (Is there malaise?)	If anorexia and malaise present, suspect malignant disease, with or without secondary spread. However, 70% of those with carcinoma of oesophagus do not have reduction in appetite, and feel well

Reason for questions	Questions asked	Comment
Neurogenic cause	Are you able to start swallowing easily? Can you make the swallowing movement easily? Have you had a stroke in the past?	Neurogenic cause may explain difficulty in initiating swallowing or making the swallowing movement
Pharyngeal pouch	Do you notice bulging or gurgling in your neck when you swallow?	Pharyngeal pouch, but accounts for less than than 1% of causes of dysphagia
Hiatus hernia, benign oesophageal stricture	Do you get heartburn, an acid taste in your mouth, or pain in the upper part of your tummy? Or pain when you lie flat or bend down?	If yes to any of these, suspect hiatus hernia and reflux as a cause of benign oesophageal stricture
Globus hystericus	Do you feel a constant lump in the throat even when you are not trying to swallow?	If yes, suspect globus hystericus, but this condition is uncommon as a cause of dysphagia
Achalasia	Are alcohol and hot drinks more or less difficult to swallow?	More difficult with a benign stricture, especially achalasia
Corrosive substances	Have you accidentally or deliberately swallowed any harmful substance?	Do not forget foreign bodies or corrosive substances, especially button batteries in children

6

Find out about complications of dysphagia	Any coughing bouts especially at night? Do you bring up a lot of phlegm or cough up blood?	May be due to regurgitation of saliva, common when oesophageal stricture severe.
Pulmonary complications	Are you unduly breathless?	May be due to aspiration pneumonia (rarely) or to secondaries in the lungs
Weight loss	Has your weight changed? If so, by how much in how long? (see Introduction for enquiry about weight loss)	Weight loss may be due to inadequate food intake or to malignancy
Pain	Does it hurt when you swallow?	Pain may be the colic of an impacted bolus, especially with malignant obstruction, or contact pain of hot, alcoholic or spicy substances in the presence of oesophagitis with a benign peptic stricture
Haematemesis/ melaena	Have you vomited blood? Have you noticed a change in the colour of your stools?	Haematemesis/melaena suggest peptic oesophagitis and hiatus hernia
Voice change	Has there been a change in your voice?	Hoarseness suggests involvement of the recurrent laryngeal nerve by malignant tumour, for instance of thyroid or oesophagus. Dysphagia as a primary symptom of carcinoma of thyroid occurs in less than 5% of patients with this disease

Reason for questions	Questions asked	Comment
ROS	Rest of GIT, CVS, RS (already included in history above), CNS, GUS	
Globus hystericus	Psychiatric history (Hope *et al.*, 1989)	If there are strong neurotic symptoms, consider globus hystericus. Also possibility of self harm by ingestion of foreign substance. Remember, however, that even people with psychiatric illness get organic disease
PMH		
Reflux during pregnancy	Ask also about reflux symptoms during pregnancy if female and previously pregnant	Symptoms of reflux occur in 75% of women asked. Reflux commoner with breech presentation. Reflux persists in less than 5% of women who did not have it before pregnancy
Heart disease	History of heart disease?	Cardiac enlargement may cause dysphagia, but very rarely
Corrosive injury	Overdoses, accidental or deliberate ingestion of caustic substances? If yes, document if possible the exact substance, the amount ingested, the concentration and the treatment given afterwards	The development of stricture after ingestion of corrosive substance depends on the substance, its concentration and quantity

Iatrogenic injury to oesophagus	History of previous surgery and use of nasogastric tubes	Traumatic stricture of the oesophagus
FH, SH, DRUGS	Some patients have a family history of carcinoma of the stomach or oesophagus. *Smoking is associated with hiatus hernia and carcinoma of the stomach and oesophagus. Alcohol often makes the pain of dysphagia worse if there is a benign stricture. Slow K is a rare cause of oesophageal stricture.* Ingestion of other cardiac drugs should alert you to the possibility of cardiac enlargement	
ALLERGIES		

Examination

Reason for examination	*Signs looked for*	*Comment*
General examination *Well-being* *Cachexia* *Spread of malignancy*	Achalasia more common in the 20–40 age group and malignancy more likely in patients aged over 65 years. Assess whether the patient is ill or well, and note the state of hydration. Look for jaundice which may indicate liver involvement by malignancy of the oesophagus or stomach. Pallor indicates anaemia; in a patient with anaemia and dysphagia think of the Patterson–Brown–Kelly syndrome; but this condition is rare. Examine for lymph node enlargement especially in the left supraclavicular fossa. An enlarged node with carcinoma of the stomach or oesophagus is Virchow's node. Its presence is Troisier's sign.	

Reason for examination	Signs looked for	Comment
Signs which suggest a cause in neck	Gurgling mass in neck	This is typical of pharyngeal pouch
	Enlarged thyroid, determine if retrosternal	Think of multinodular goitre or carcinoma as a cause of dysphagia
Look for signs of oropharyngeal infection	Examine mouth, tonsils and pharynx. Oral candidiasis, tonsillitis and other oropharyngeal infections can cause dysphagia.	
Finish rest of general examination		
Systematic examination *Lung involvement*	RS: Reduced chest wall movement, dullness to percussion, bronchial breathing and crackles suggest secondaries or rarely aspiration pneumonia. Note, however, that there may be no RS findings even with widespread lung secondaries.	
	CVS examination: heart enlargement can cause dysphagia as mentioned above.	
Abdominal examination looking for features of malignancy	There may be scars from previous operations. Were such operations for malignancy?	
	Examine for ascites (Browse, 1993) but note that small amounts are difficult to detect. If ascites present there is a strong possibility of carcinoma of the oesophagus or stomach.	
	If a mass is present, is it due to carcinoma of the stomach?	

	Hepatomegaly should raise the possibility of secondary carcinoma or heart failure with cardiomegaly.
	Rectal and vaginal examination: if a mass found in the Pouch of Douglas in a woman, think of Krukenberg tumour from a primary in stomach. It is rare.
	Finish rest of abdominal examination.
CNS	Neurological signs in a patient with dysphagia should make you think of bulbar palsy, myasthenia gravis, or secondary carcinoma.
Psychiatric examination (Hope *et al.*, 1989)	Globus hystericus must be considered in a patient with neurotic symptoms but you must first rule out organic disease.

Investigations

The order of investigation will depend on the disease suspected.

Benign oesophageal stricture

Barium swallow and upper gastrointestinal endoscopy to confirm diagnosis and reveal cause.

Additional investigations: full blood count, chest X-ray.

Carcinoma of the oesophagus or stomach

Barium swallow and meal and upper gastrointestinal endoscopy and biopsy to confirm diagnosis.

LFTs, chest X-ray, ultrasound of the abdomen to assess whether tumour has spread to liver or lungs.

FBC to determine if anaemia present.

11

Foreign body in the oesophagus

Plain X-ray of the neck and chest may show a radio-opaque foreign body. Look for subcutaneous emphysema in neck if oesophageal rupture likely. Radiolucent foreign bodies do not show on plain X-ray.

When indicated, oesophagoscopy will show foreign body and allow its removal.

Achalasia of oesophagus

Barium swallow and upper gastrointestinal endoscopy.

Additional investigations: full blood count, oesophageal manometry and chest X-ray.

Interpretation of tests in dysphagia

Urinalysis for bilirubin: The presence of urinary bilirubin suggests intrahepatic obstruction due to secondaries from carcinoma.

Faecal occult blood: This test is of value if dysphagia presents with iron deficiency anaemia, for it indicates either a hiatus hernia which is bleeding or the Patterson–Brown–Kelly syndrome.

More often the test is performed when anaemia is found and the cause is unclear.

Haemoglobin: Anaemia suggests carcinoma or a bleeding hiatus hernia.

U&Es: These may be deranged in the presence of dehydration from inadequate fluid intake.

LFTs: Abnormal LFTs suggest secondaries in the liver from carcinoma of the oesophagus or stomach.

Chest X-ray: This should be done in all patients with dysphagia to determine whether or not there is aspiration pneumonia, secondary carcinoma or cardiac enlargement. Also, achalasia may show as a dilated upper oesophagus on the plain film. Hiatus hernia may show as a large gas shadow with a fluid level on the lower part of the chest X-ray.

X-ray of thoracic inlet: Important if the thyroid is found to be enlarged and extends retrosternally. It may show deviation of the trachea.

Barium swallow: The radiologist must be given enough information to enable him to adapt the investigation to the patient's problem. This X-ray will show the site and nature of a stricture, and the completeness of obstruction.

The calibre of the oesophagus above the lesion will also be shown.

Lesions which often show characteristic features are carcinoma and achalasia.

Hiatus hernias are commonly demonstrated even in patients with no symptoms. Reflux of barium into the oesophagus is also demonstrated but this does not give any information about whether the reflux is pathological.

Upper gastrointestinal endoscopy: This is mandatory in all patients with dysphagia, for it will allow direct visualization of the abnormal area and enable biopsies and brushings to be taken for histological and cytological examination. Reflux oesophagitis can also be assessed and the mucosa of the stomach and duodenum inspected.

Bronchoscopy: Will be necessary if the cause of the dysphagia is thought to be carcinoma of the bronchus.

Ultrasound of the liver: Is useful if secondary carcinoma of the liver is suspected.

Oesophageal manometry: The pressures in the oesophagus and the motility pattern of the oesophageal muscle will be determined. In achalasia the lowermost segment of the oesophagus fails to relax when a wave of peristalsis reaches it.

Case report

Features	Analysis
Mrs Jane Smith is 75 years of age and has had difficulty swallowing solid foods for 4 months.	Dysphagia of recent onset in a patient aged 75 should immediately alert you to the possibility of carcinoma of the oesophagus or upper stomach. However, you must keep an open mind until you have considered all the information available.
This lady was well and free of symptoms until 4 months ago when she experienced difficulty with swallowing. It started one night when she went out for a meal with her husband to celebrate their 50th wedding anniversary. She had ordered a plate of steak and chips, and noticed that when she tried her first mouthful of meat, it seemed to stick in the mid-sternal region. She had pain behind the sternum but it cleared after she drank a large glass of water. She did not tell her husband about this at the time and managed to finish that meal by chewing every morsel for as long as possible.	A detailed history of the onset and progression of dysphagia is important. In this case it started suddenly and progressed without remission to the point where she could swallow only semi-solids and liquids. Benign and malignant strictures of the oesophagus and carcinoma of the cardia can produce these features.

This problem persisted for the next 4 months and she decided to seek medical advice when she found that solids, however well chewed, would not go down. They stuck always at the mid-sternal level. As she could no longer swallow solids, she avoided them. She could swallow semi-solid foods such as porridge if she ate them slowly, and could swallow liquids easily.

The type of food the patient can swallow does not tell you much about the underlying condition, but gives some information about nutritional deficit. Inability to swallow liquids and saliva is due to severe obstruction of the oesophagus.

On three occasions in the previous 3 months she regurgitated the food she ate. Her husband had noticed that several times in the night for the last 2 months, she would wake him up with the noise of her persistent coughing and choking.

Regurgitation does not tell you about the cause of dysphagia, merely its severity. It occurs when the calibre of the oesophagus is reduced to the point where the food eaten stagnates above the obstruction.

Choking and coughing at night suggest spillage of oesophageal contents into the air passages, again suggesting severe oesophageal narrowing.

Her appetite was good and she had managed to maintain her weight by drinking lots of nutritious liquids such as Complan, and she felt well in herself.

Maintenance of appetite and weight does not rule out malignancy. This lady has altered her eating pattern to make sure she does not lose weight.

When she sat down to eat, she could start swallowing easily and could make the swallowing movement when not eating. She did not get bulging or a gurgling in her neck. She did not feel a constant lump in her throat when she was not trying to swallow.

Think of other causes of dysphagia such as neurogenic disturbance and globus hystericus. A negative history does not rule them out.

Features	*Analysis*
For the last 5 years she suffered from epigastric pain and heartburn made worse by lying flat and bending over to pick things up. She did not drink alcohol and had never deliberately or accidentally swallowed any harmful substances. She had never vomited blood nor noticed a change in the colour of her stools. There had been no change in her voice.	This suggests a hiatus hernia, raising the possibility that the oesophageal obstruction is secondary to reflux. Remember, however, that symptoms of hiatus hernia can be obtained in as many as 30% of patients of this age who prove to have carcinoma of the oesophagus.
She never had jaundice or pain in her abdomen other than the epigastric pain mentioned above. Her bowels were regular and her stools normal.	
There were no other symptoms on systems review other than pain from osteoarthritis of both hips for which she took paracetamol. She was not taking any other medications and there was nothing remarkable in her family and social history.	
On examination, she looked well and was not anaemic or jaundiced. Her head, neck, axillae and breasts were normal. There were no lymph nodes in the cervical or supraclavicular regions. She was normotensive and her heart and lungs were normal. There were no abnormal findings in the abdomen. The liver was not palpable and there were no masses in the abdomen. Hernial orifices were intact and rectal and vaginal examinations were normal. She had varicose veins in the region of the great saphenous vein in both legs but there were no ulcers. All pulses were palpable and were normal.	It is not surprising for physical signs to be absent in dysphagia from most causes. Features of malignancy are present in many cases if the tumour is advanced. Nevertheless, thorough examination is important to ensure that the patient is fully assessed. This lady was found to have varicose veins, which are almost certainly unrelated to her dysphagia.

| Neurological examination did not reveal any abnormalities. | Neurological examination is important. Positive findings suggest either a neurological cause for the dysphagia, for instance bulbar palsy, or metastatic disease to the brain from oesophageal or gastric cancer. |

Clinical diagnosis

The two most likely diagnoses in this lady are carcinoma of the oesophagus or cardia and benign oesophageal stricture due to reflux. In favour of carcinoma are her age, the recent onset of dysphagia and its relentless progression. Do not be put off this diagnosis by her good appetite, maintenance of her normal weight, her apparent good health and the absence of features such as anaemia and jaundice. Benign stricture is suggested by the 5-year history of epigastric pain and heartburn, followed by dysphagia. Many of the other items in the history indicate that the oesophagus has become progressively narrowed, but do not tell us much about the cause. You must think of the other possible causes of dysphagia such as carcinoma of the bronchus and foreign bodies but there is little in the history to support them.

Investigations and final diagnosis

| Barium swallow showed a malignant looking obstruction of the middle third of the oesophagus. The obstruction was not complete and contrast flowed into the lower oesophagus and stomach to demonstrate a sliding hiatus hernia. | There were features in the history to suggest both lesions, and investigation showed them both to be present. This demonstrates the value of good history and examination. |
| At oesophagoscopy this lesion looked malignant. Biopsy showed a squamous carcinoma. | Upper GIT endoscopy is mandatory in almost all patients with dysphagia, unless, as mentioned above, an obvious lesion such as tonsillitis is the cause. |

Features	Analysis
Her Hb was 12.5 g/dl, WCC 9.5x10⁹/l. U&Es and LFTs, including albumin, were normal.	Normal LFTs do not rule out secondaries in the liver. The liver has an enormous reserve capacity.
Chest X-ray was clear but ultrasound of the liver showed two suspicious lesions which proved at operation to be metastatic deposits from the primary tumour in the oesophagus.	Despite her night coughs, her chest X-ray was normal. The secondary deposits in the liver, though not predicted from the clinical findings and blood tests, were not surprising. Only 10% of livers with secondaries are detectable on clinical examination.

References

Browse, N. (1993) *An introduction to the Symptoms and Signs of Surgical Disease* (second edition). Edward Arnold, London.

Hobsley, M. (1989) *Pathways in Surgical Management* (third edition). Edward Arnold, London, pp. 83–94.

Hope, R. A., Longmore, J. M., Hodgetts, T. J., Ramrakha, P. S. (1994) *Oxford Handbook of Clinical Medicine* (third edition). Oxford University Press, Oxford.

Chapter 2

Non-acute or recurrent upper abdominal pain

The pain is usually of more than a week's duration and is not sufficiently severe to warrant admission to hospital. It is one of the commonest reasons for patients seeking consultation with surgeons. In many practices, up to two-thirds of patients presenting with such pain do not have a demonstrable abnormality. There is an enormous overlap between the symptoms of diseases from different organs, and in making a diagnosis it is important to take all the evidence available, rather than rely on a few seemingly characteristic features.

Causes

Anatomical classification

Based on the organ in which the pain has arisen.
(a) Oesophagus
    (i) Reflux oesophagitis

(b) Stomach
    (i) Gastric ulcer
    (ii) Gastric carcinoma
    (iii) Gastritis
(c) Duodenum
    (i) Duodenal ulcer
    (ii) Duodenitis
(d) Liver
    (i) Hepatitis
    (ii) Liver tumours, primary and secondary
    (iii) Heart failure (distension of the liver capsule)
    (iv) Infestations of the liver, e.g. hydatid disease
    (v) Liver abscess
(e) Biliary tract
    (i) Stone in the gall bladder, cystic duct, common bile duct
    (ii) Cholecystitis, with or without stones

(f) Pancreas
   (i) Chronic pancreatitis
   (ii) Carcinoma of the pancreas

Commoner causes

Peptic ulcer (gastric and duodenal ulcer) (40%), gall stones (20%), reflux oesophagitis (10%), carcinoma of the stomach (5%), chronic pancreatitis (5%), carcinoma of the pancreas (3%).

Points to look for

Gastric and duodenal ulcer

Difficult to distinguish between the two from history and examination alone, despite claims in some older books.

Pain located in the epigastrium and occurs shortly after a meal or when patient is hungry, and is relieved by food (especially milk) or alkalis.

It is common for the pain to wake the patient up in the early hours of the morning. 85% of patients with peptic ulcer complain of pain occurring during the night.

Symptoms are periodic in 90%: typically they occur for about 4 weeks, ease for 9–12 months and are likely to recur.

Gall stones

Occur in both sexes and at any age, not just in the 'fair, fat, fertile, flatulent female of forty'.

Commoner in women and prevalence increases with increasing age. By the age of 70 years it is estimated that 15% of people have gall stones. However, many stones are asymptomatic, and merely finding them does not mean that they are the cause of the patient's symptoms.

Pain intermittent and lasts from a few hours to several days.

During an attack, pain varies in intensity.

There may be nausea and vomiting.

Pain located usually in the right hypochondrium (90%) but may be anywhere in the upper abdomen; it may radiate to the back or the tip of the right shoulder.

In between or instead of acute attacks, the
patient complains of mild epigastric discomfort
with abdominal distension and belching of
wind.

Reflux oesophagitis

20% of patients with reflux oesophagitis are
obese.

Main feature is heartburn on lying flat or
stooping forwards.

Pain starts in epigastrium and radiates upwards
behind the sternum.

Smoking aggravates symptoms.

Dysphagia in such a patient suggests
development of stricture of the oesophagus.

Note that many patients with hiatus hernia do
not have reflux; 20% of patients with reflux do
not have a hiatus hernia; and reflux can be
present without oesophagitis.

Carcinoma of stomach

Discussed in chapter on dysphagia. Up to 60% of
patients with carcinoma of stomach do not
have pain as a presenting symptom, but on
direct questioning, 95% will admit to pain.
When pain is present, it is difficult to
distinguish from benign peptic ulcer.

Anorexia and weight loss present in 25% of
patients at first presentation.

Carcinoma of pancreas

Does not produce symptoms until far advanced
in 55%.

85% of patients in whom this diagnosis has been
made admit to pain in the back. It is worse on
lying flat and relieved by sitting up and
bending forward. This characteristic pain is
also produced by chronic pancreatitis; but only
10% of patients with carcinoma of the
pancreas or chronic pancreatitis have this
typical pain.

60% of patients in whom carcinoma of the head
of the pancreas is diagnosed present with
painless obstructive jaundice as the sole
symptom.

Chronic pancreatitis

Pain often located in the epigastrium and made
worse by lying flat and by ingestion of alcohol.
May radiate to the back.

There is a history of alcohol abuse in 40%,
steatorrhoea in 10%, and diabetes mellitus
in 5%.

History

Reason for question	*Question asked*	*Comment*
Site and radiation of pain	Please can you show me where you get the pain? When the pain gets worse, where else does it go, or where else do you feel the pain?	The site to which the patient points may help in diagnosis: Right hypochondrium radiating to back or shoulder tip: – gall bladder disease Epigastric pain radiating to the middle of the back: – chronic pancreatitis, pancreatic carcinoma, penetrating duodenal ulcer Epigastric pain radiating behind the sternum: – reflux oesophagitis

Severity of pain	How does this pain affect your life? (effect on work, leisure, personal relationships, sleep)	Individual thresholds are different for the same pain, and the patient may exaggerate or minimize his pain. A more accurate way of assessing severity of pain is to determine its effect on the patient's life. A patient may describe the pain as severe and yet go to work or to the pub while he has it. *The severity of a pain does not give any reliable clues as to cause or underlying disease, but it is of great importance when deciding how to treat the patient*
Mode of onset of pain and its progression	*When did the pain first start?* How did it start? *How has it progressed since?* Is it getting better or worse, or is it staying about the same? Is it coming on more or less frequently? How often do you get the pain? How many times a day (or week, month, year)? When the pain comes, describe to me exactly what happens, what you do, what you take? How does the pain end? *How long does the pain take to subside?*	Again, these questions do not elicit cause but give an indication of the severity or of the persistent character of the pain. It will give the patient a chance to describe the pain without leading questions Gall bladder pain may take several hours to subside The pain from carcinoma of the stomach is more or less continuous, and is often made worse by food. Pain from chronic pancreatitis is sometimes continuous

Reason for question	Question asked	Comment
Nature of pain	Please describe the pain to me. *When it comes, is it there all of the time, or does it come and go in waves? Are you completely free of pain in between attacks, or do you feel a background ache?* Is it aching, stabbing, throbbing or burning? Does the pain make you roll around or does it make you lie still?	True colic, namely pain which is recurring and griping in nature, with complete freedom from pain in between bouts, occurs in obstruction of any hollow viscus. When due to intestinal obstruction, it is very characteristic, and can be diagnosed from the patient's story. It starts gradually, builds up to a peak and then dies away ('like green apples going through'). It lasts about 2 or 3 minutes, and may recur within about 20 minutes. The patient rolls around when the pain gets severe. Think of obstructive causes in the lumen, in the wall and outside the wall of the bowel. Biliary 'colic' lasts about 30 minutes, renal 'colic' about 20 minutes, but there are wide variations
Precipitating factors and aggravating factors. Food	What brings the pain on? Food?	Pain of gastric ulcer is brought on by food, and hence the patient is afraid to eat Pain of gall bladder disease comes on a few hours after food but it is not thought to be any worse after fats

		The pain of hiatus hernia is associated with taking food and relieved by belching
		Lack of food often brings on the pain of duodenal ulcer (hunger pain) and eating relieves it. However, the reverse may be true and it not possible to distinguish between gastric ulcer and duodenal ulcer from this
Drink	Does drink bring the pain on? What sorts of drinks?	Pain due to gastric ulcer, gastritis, hiatus hernia and duodenal ulcer is brought on and aggravated by alcoholic beverages
Posture	Is the pain brought on by any positions you lie in? What positions?	Pain of hiatus hernia is characteristically brought on by lying flat in bed and also by bending over, for instance to tie shoe laces. The pain of pancreatitis also tends to occur when the patient lies flat and is sometimes eased by sitting up and bending forwards
Others/drugs	Do you know of anything else that brings your pain on?	Some drugs such as NSAIDs and steroids aggravate the pain of gastric ulcer and gastric erosions
Relieving factors Vomiting	What makes the pain better? Vomiting?	The pain of gall bladder disease, gastric ulcer and gastric cancer is often relieved by vomiting

Reason for question	Question asked	Comment
Food	Food?	Duodenal ulcer pain improved by food, but see notes above
Belching	Belching?	Belching makes the pain of hiatus hernia better
Associated features	Does the pain wake you up at night?	The pain of hiatus hernia occurs when the patient slips into the supine position at night. The pain of peptic ulcer wakes the patient up at about 2 a.m. when the volume of resting acid juice in the stomach is high
	What do you think is the cause of your pain?	The patient may well have recognized an association between the pain and some event which you have not thought about. It is worth making a note of any information the patient gives you
ROS	*Rest of GIT:* What is your appetite like? Has there been any change in your weight? (see Introduction for enquiry into weight loss)	Poor appetite and weight loss should alert you to the possibility of malignant disease, especially of the stomach and pancreas and of secondaries in the liver. These symptoms can also occur in duodenal ulcer which is progressing to pyloric stenosis. They are characteristic of gastric ulcer in which the patient does not eat for fear of precipitating pain

Do you have any difficulty swallowing?	If yes, make further enquiry as described in the chapter on dysphagia. The presence of dysphagia suggests carcinoma of the oesophagus or stomach, or a benign stricture of the oesophagus following oesophagitis
Do you get a sickly feeling? Do you vomit? How much, how often?	Vomiting suggests carcinoma of the stomach or gastric ulcer; it also occurs with psychogenic pain
What do you vomit?	If the vomitus is bile stained the pylorus is probably not obstructed. Blood in the vomit may be due to ulceration of the oesophagus, stomach or duodenum
Do you belch a lot of wind?	Occurs with hiatus hernia and gall bladder disease
Have you had jaundice?	Hepatitis, secondary carcinoma, gall stones, pancreatitis, pancreatic carcinoma
Does your tummy bloat or swell up?	Pyloric stenosis, gall bladder disease, malignant tumours in the abdomen, ascites
What are your bowels like? Has there been a change? What are the motions like?	Diarrhoea and steatorrhoea may be due to chronic pancreatitis
RS Cough, sputum, haemoptysis, dyspnoea?	Secondary carcinoma, pulmonary infections due to aspiration in dysphagia. Pain from pulmonary disease can be referred to the abdomen

Reason for question	Question asked	Comment
CVS	Angina?	Ischaemic cardiac pain can be referred to the abdomen
	Palpitations, orthopnoea, paroxysmal nocturnal dyspnoea, ankle swellings?	Congestive cardiac failure can cause hepatic pain due to distension of its capsule
	CNS, GUS, PSYCHIATRIC HISTORY	

PMH	**If:**
	Previous laparotomy
	Previous operation for cancer
	                    peptic ulcer
	                    gall stones
		Think of:
		Intestinal adhesions, incisional hernia
		Recurrence or secondaries
		Recurrent or stomal ulcer
		Recurrent or residual stones

FH	Peptic ulcer, cancer, heart disease	
SH	Smoking	Cancer, peptic ulcer, heart disease
	Alcohol	Pancreatitis, peptic ulcer, liver damage
	Trips abroad	Hydatid disease, liver abscess, hepatitis
DRUGS	Steroids, aspirin, NSAIDs	Peptic ulcer, gastritis
	Antacids, anti-ulcer drugs	Known ulcer disease
ALLERGIES		

Examination

Reason for examination	Signs looked for	Comment
General examination	The patient may look ill, wasted and anaemic with neoplasia, but as mentioned above, this is rarely the case. Patients may also lose weight with gastric ulcer and chronic pancreatitis. Secondary carcinoma, obstruction of the biliary tree by tumour within it or in the pancreas, stones or chronic pancreatitis, and hepatitis may all result in obstructive jaundice.	
	Lymph node enlargement (examine the neck, supraclavicular fossae, axillae and inguinal areas)	If present, suspect carcinoma, especially of the pancreas and stomach
RS	Signs of infection, collapse, consolidation, pleural effusion	Suggest secondary carcinoma from a primary in pancreas or stomach
CVS		Congestive cardiac failure may cause an enlarged, tender liver
CNS		Secondary carcinoma in the brain may cause raised intracranial pressure and focal neurological deficits such as weakness or sensory loss (rare with carcinoma of stomach)

Reason for examination	Signs looked for	Comment
ABDOMEN	Inspection: Scars	Previous operations (see past medical history); adhesions;
	Incisional hernias	May cause abdominal wall pain
	Distension	With an abdominal mass or ascites, suspect carcinoma of the stomach. Ascites may be due to portal hypertension
	Palpation:	The gall bladder and a tumour in the stomach may be palpable. An enlarged liver may be due to secondaries or congestive cardiac failure
	Percussion:	Shifting dullness in ascites. Dullness over a mass or enlarged liver
	Auscultation:	
	Gastric succussion splash	Pyloric obstruction from gastric tumour or scarring due to duodenal ulcer
Rest of abdominal examination	Examine the groins, genitalia and rectum Examine the back	
LOWER LIMBS		

Investigations

The investigation carried out depends on the disease suspected.

Gall stones

Ultrasound of the upper abdomen is the commonest method of diagnosing gall stones.

Other tests: plain X-ray of the abdomen, liver function tests, oral cholecystogram, ERCP.

Gastric and duodenal ulcer

Barium meal; upper gastrointestinal endoscopy to allow visualization of the ulcer and biopsy.

Other tests: blood count.

Reflux oesophagitis

Upper gastrointestinal endoscopy, barium meal.

Other tests: blood count, plain X-ray of the chest (may show a hiatus hernia), pH measurement in oesophagus.

Carcinoma of stomach

Barium meal, upper gastrointestinal endoscopy, blood count, ESR.

Other tests: chest X-ray, ultrasound of the liver, liver function tests.

Carcinoma of the pancreas

Ultrasound and CT scan of the abdomen, ERCP, needle biopsy under CT guidance. Even with these facilities, the diagnosis of this condition is notoriously difficult.

Chronic pancreatitis

Plain X-ray of the abdomen may show speckled pancreatic calcification; blood glucose (diabetes); ERCP; CT scan and ultrasound of the abdomen.

Case report

Features	*Analysis*
Mrs June Bloggs is 38 years old. She presented with an 18-month history of pain in the epigastrium radiating retrosternally. Sometimes the pain radiated to her back to between the shoulder blades. There were no precipitating factors but her symptoms were much worse when she lay flat or bent over, for example to pick up her 3-year-old child. She was also frequently woken up from sleep by the pain and had to drink milk to get relief. The pain was also a little easier when she belched. She complained that her abdomen bloated and this made her bring up a lot of wind.	Gastro-oesophageal reflux is the most likely cause of this lady's symptoms. The site of the pain, its radiation retrosternally, and its relation to posture suggest this diagnosis. However, there are features which make it imperative to consider other diagnoses: radiation to between the shoulder blades, belching and abdominal distension (gall bladder disease); waking up with the pain in the early hours of the morning (peptic ulcer). These conditions must be investigated.
She denied dysphagia, regurgitation or vomiting and had not noticed any change in the colour of her stools. She had not had jaundice.	Enquire into complications of reflux such as oesophageal stricture or bleeding from oesophagitis. Jaundice may be due to gall stones and haematemesis/melaena may complicate peptic ulcer.
When questioned, she admitted that she had had similar symptoms in her previous two pregnancies but they improved after delivery. This time the pain had started 18 months after the last pregnancy. She was not pregnant at this presentation.	Many women get reflux symptoms during pregnancy, but such symptoms regress in the majority.

She did not smoke and drank 7 units of alcohol a week. She had tried a variety of antacids and most did not make much difference to her heartburn. She had had no major illnesses and had not undergone any operations.

Smoking exacerbates the symptoms of reflux oesophagitis and delays healing of peptic ulcer.

On examination she was well, though moderately obese. She was not anaemic. Heart and lungs were normal. Abdominal examination did not reveal any abnormalities. The remainder of the examination was normal.

A complete lack of physical findings apart from obesity is common in all the conditions under investigation.

Clinical diagnosis

As mentioned above, this lady probably has gastro-oesophageal reflux but must be investigated for peptic ulcer and gall stones. The features in favour of these possible diagnoses are discussed in the analysis.

Investigations

Upper gastrointestinal endoscopy showed an inflamed lower oesophageal mucosa with multiple erosions. Biopsies were taken from this area. There was no evidence of hiatus hernia. The endoscope could be passed easily into the stomach.

The stomach and duodenum were normal.

These are the endoscopic features of oesophagitis.

This condition can occur even in the absence of a hiatus hernia. It was important to exclude a coexisting peptic ulcer.

Barium meal showed neither an oesophageal stricture nor a hiatus hernia.

Stricture is an important complication of oesophagitis and must be looked for.

33

Features	Analysis
24-hour pH measurement showed several episodes in the day when the pH in the lower oesophagus fell to below 4, confirming reflux.	
Ultrasound of the upper abdomen did not show any abnormalities in the liver, gall bladder, bile ducts or pancreas.	Some of this lady's symptoms were suggestive of gall bladder disease; so it was important to do an ultrasound examination of the upper abdomen.

Final diagnosis
Gastro-oesophageal reflux not associated with hiatus hernia and not complicated by oesophageal stricture.

Chapter 3

Acute abdominal pain

Much work has been done in the last 15 years to clarify the diagnosis of acute abdominal pain. A team of researchers, headed by Professor Tim de Dombal in Leeds, England, has done more than any other to promote our understanding of this condition. Most of the information presented here has been obtained from their work. I recommend de Dombal's book on acute abdominal pain (see Reference list).

Definition

Acute abdominal pain is defined as undiagnosed abdominal pain present for less than a week and severe enough for the patient to seek help from his doctor. Two conditions excluded are abdominal trauma and obviously strangulated hernia. I will not cover the former but will discuss the latter, which is often overlooked by students.

Underlying pathology

When you diagnose the cause of abdominal pain, you must attempt to do two things: (A) decide on the organ or system affected and (B) determine the disease process in that organ. For example, *acute cholecystitis* means that the gall bladder is the organ and the disease affecting it is infection or inflammation. Every organ in the abdomen and many outside it cause abdominal pain, but as we shall see below, those most commonly affected are few.

Traditionally, it is taught that in most cases, there are three basic disease processes that affect an organ to cause abdominal pain: (a) the organ (a hollow viscus) can become obstructed; (b) an organ can become inflamed or (c) it can perforate.

The pain resulting from (a) is visceral pain and is termed 'colic'; it will frequently be referred to the appropriate dermatome. It may, therefore, be felt at a site well away from the viscus. The pain from (b) is due to inflammation involving the local peritoneum and localizes over the viscus. The pain from (c) is more widespread, and may be all over the abdomen. Each of these pathological processes has distinct clinical features.

What makes this classification difficult for the student initially is that more than one of these pathological states may be present in an organ. For instance, acute appendicitis may start with colicky pain around the centre of the abdomen (visceral pain). Later, the pain localizes in the right lower quadrant, where there is tenderness and muscle guarding (peritoneal inflammation). If the disease progresses, the appendix may perforate and cause generalized peritonitis. Some patients present at phase (b) without having recognized phase (a), or even at phase (c) without any of the previous phases being apparent. This classification is an oversimplification, but is of clinical value, as seen below.

(a) Colic

The characteristics of colic have been described in Chapter 2. One feature of colic, which distinguishes it from intraperitoneal inflammation or infection, is that when colic occurs, the patient cannot lie still and is constantly moving in an attempt to find a comfortable position. True colic occurs in intestinal obstruction.

(b) Local peritonitis

On the other hand, with intraperitoneal inflammation, movement such as coughing or deep breathing produces friction between the inflamed surfaces of the peritoneum, and hence the patient tends to lie still. Examination reveals tenderness, muscle guarding, rigidity and rebound tenderness, localized in the part of the abdomen affected. The rest of the abdomen is soft, with little or no tenderness. Bowel sounds are often normal.

(c) Generalized peritonitis

The pain may have started as visceral pain, progressing to local peritonitis, and then to general peritonitis. In many cases, such a distinct progression is not recognized by the patient, who may be pain free one minute and then have generalized abdominal pain the next. The patient is in pain, he looks ill and dehydrated, and has general abdominal tenderness, muscle guarding and rigidity, and rebound tenderness. Bowel sounds will be absent a few hours after the onset of the pain in many cases.

Does the patient need resuscitation?

Acute abdominal pain is an emergency, and the first priority is to decide whether the patient requires resuscitation. If the patient is shocked or dehydrated, insert an intravenous cannula, obtain blood for haemoglobin, PCV, WCC, U&Es, amylase and glucose, and also for grouping and cross matching. The number of units of blood requested depends on the initial diagnostic impression. If, for instance, perforated duodenal ulcer is suspected, 2 units of whole blood would suffice. On the other hand, if a leaking aortic aneurysm is thought likely, ask for at least 6 units of blood. If the patient is bleeding, clotting screening and platelet count should also be performed. Start an intravenous infusion as soon as blood has been obtained for tests.

Are analgesics required?

Analgesics are often withheld from patients with acute abdominal pain because these drugs are believed to mask signs. Research shows that they do not. On the contrary, in some cases, they make it easier to examine the patient. Once a good working diagnosis is made, an analgesic drug must be administered without delay to all except those with mild pain.

Causes of acute abdominal pain

There are numerous causes of acute abdominal pain. As mentioned above, some causes are in the abdomen and others outside. A long list of causes is more likely to confuse. What is more useful is to consider the commonest causes presenting to the emergency unit.

Non-specific abdominal pain

In approximately 55% of patients presenting with acute abdominal pain, no definite cause is found even after extensive investigation. These patients are said to suffer from 'non-specific abdominal pain' (NSAP).

The student must realize that this is not a diagnosis, and some authorities argue that this term is an expression of our ignorance. Nonetheless, it is a useful term which denotes that such patients do not have any of the recognizable causes of acute abdominal pain, and equally importantly, they do not need an operation. Do not use this term merely because a diagnosis has not been made. Even experienced clinicians do not always get the diagnosis right.

Commoner causes of acute abdominal pain

Non-specific abdominal pain (55%), acute appendicitis (18%), acute cholecystitis (7%), urinary tract disorders (mainly ureteric calculi) (6%), gynaecological problems (5%), small bowel obstruction (3%), perforated peptic ulcer (3%), acute pancreatitis (2%) (Wilson *et al.*, 1977).

Less common but important causes

Malignant disease (especially carcinoma of colon) ($<1\%$), diverticular disease ($<1\%$), mesenteric vascular occlusion ($<1\%$), leaking aortic aneurysm ($<1\%$), obstructed or strangulated hernia ($<1\%$).

These proportions increase about 5-fold in patients over 50 years of age.

Special categories of patients

In women of childbearing age, the commonest causes of acute abdominal pain are NSAP (50%), appendicitis (20%), pelvic inflammatory disease (15%), complications of ovarian cyst (12%).

Ectopic pregnancy accounts for only 1% but is an important diagnosis to bear in mind (Walmsley *et al.*, 1977).

In patients over the age of 50: see above.

In children under the age of 10, appendicitis (30%), NSAP (60%), urinary infection (2%), intussusception (1.5%) (Dickson *et al.*, 1988).

Points to look for

Acute appendicitis

Commonest between the ages of 10 and 30 years (60%

of cases) and slightly more common in males than females.

Classically, the pain starts as colic in the centre of the abdomen and later localizes in the right lower quadrant. Note, however, that at the time of presentation, only 75% of patients have right lower quadrant pain. The rest have pain in the centre or across the lower abdomen.

In over 50%, pain aggravated by coughing or movement.

Anorexia, nausea and vomiting present in most patients with appendicitis but these symptoms occur in other conditions. Absence of these symptoms makes appendicitis less likely but does not rule it out.

Facial flushing without pyrexia strongly suggests appendicitis. Characteristic abdominal findings are focal tenderness, guarding and rebound tenderness in the right lower quadrant.

Tenderness on the right (but not the left) side of the rectum strongly in favour of diagnosis.

Acute cholecystitis

A past history of cholecystitis or symptomatic gall stones (Chapter 2) useful in diagnosis. However, over 90% of patients with gall stones do not have symptoms. Localized, intermittent pain in the right upper quadrant of the abdomen highly suggestive of cholecystitis. Fifty percent of patients with this diagnosis have pain at this site. Another typical feature is radiation of pain to the right infrascapular region of the back. The pain is made worse by inspiration. A history of jaundice with pale stools and dark urine suggests obstruction of the common bile duct by a calculus. Typically, there is tenderness and muscle guarding in the right upper quadrant, and Murphy's sign is positive (see below). If a tender mass is found, think of empyema of the gall bladder.

To elicit Murphy's sign, you ask the patient to take a deep breath while you palpate over the region of the gall bladder. As the inflamed gall bladder descends, it comes in contact with the ridge made by your finger, and the patient's breath is caught at the height of inspiration.

Ureteric calculus and urinary tract infection

These are discussed in Chapter 11.

Pointers to gynaecological disorder in a woman with acute abdominal pain

If woman under 40, pelvic inflammatory disease more likely; if over 40, think of complication of ovarian cyst (torsion, bleeding). Pain outside the right lower quadrant, especially if bilateral, suggests gynaecological disease. Radiation of pain to shoulder tips and fainting or loss of consciousness suggest intra-abdominal bleeding, more common in ruptured ectopic pregnancy, but seen in bleeding ovarian cyst. Radiation to the thigh or back more likely with gynaecological disorders such as ectopic pregnancy, incomplete abortion and pelvic inflammatory disease than with non-gynaecological conditions such as appendicitis. Other features include vaginal discharge, a period of amenorrhoea, abnormal bleeding and dyspareunia, but their absence by no means excludes gynaecological conditions.

Think of the Fitz–Hugh–Curtis syndrome in a sexually active woman who presents with features of acute cholecystitis, especially if X-rays and scans do not reveal gall stones. In this condition, there is perihepatitis caused by chlamydia and other organisms.

Intestinal obstruction

Intestinal obstruction is rare under the age of 5 but common at all other ages. The underlying cause depends on the patient's age: intussusception in the paediatric age group; malignancy, diverticular disease and pseudo-obstruction in those over 65 years. Adhesions and hernia can cause obstruction at any age. The classic pain of intestinal obstruction is in the centre of the abdomen in 40% of patients and is colicky. Nausea, vomiting and anorexia are present in almost all patients. A history of change in bowel habit should alert you to bowel malignancy. As obstruction progresses, pain and constitutional distress increase. Look for abdominal scars, which suggest adhesions. The degree of abdominal distension increases the more distal the site of obstruction. Listen for high pitched, continuous bowel sounds and do not forget to examine hernial orifices.

Perforated peptic ulcer

More common in middle-aged men. Half the patients have a history of epigastric pain. Pain occurs suddenly, is continuous and becomes widespread with time. It is aggravated by movement, coughing and inspiration. The patient is ill, is in severe pain and lies still. The abdomen is rigid and tender, usually all over, and silent.

Acute pancreatitis

The clinical features depend on the severity of pancreatitis and the cause. They vary from mild to severe abdominal pain with profound hypotension. This disease occurs more commonly in adults: men who develop the disease are usually aged between 30 and 50 years (usually caused by alcohol) and women are aged 50–70 (gall stones).

There may have been previous attacks of acute pancreatitis. A heavy intake of alcohol before the onset of pain is relevant. In the patient whose pancreatitis is due to gall stones there may be a history of bouts of mild upper abdominal pain, abdominal distension, flatulence, nausea, and jaundice with the passage of pale stools and dark urine. Enquiry should be made about drugs such as steroids, the oral contraceptive pill, thiazide diuretics and frusemide, known to cause acute pancreatitis.

The pain often occurs suddenly, but takes some minutes to reach a peak. It is most commonly in the upper abdomen, but may be in one or other hypochondrium, or even in the lower abdomen. It spreads gradually to involve the whole abdomen, but sometimes it may remain localized. In about 50% of patients the pain radiates to the middle of the lower thoracic or upper lumbar region of the back. The pain, sometimes severe, is aggravated by movement and coughing. Some patients get relief by sitting up and bending forward, presumably to remove the pressure exerted on the pancreas by intra-abdominal organs. Nausea and vomiting occur in about 90% of patients, and in some there is haematemesis.

On examination, the patient may be well but sometimes is ill, dehydrated or shocked, jaundiced, and pyrexial. The absence of these signs does not exclude pancreatitis. Rarely, there is discoloration of the flanks (Grey–Turner's sign) or of the umbilicus (Cullen's sign). The abdomen is mildly distended and tympanitic, due to ileus. Tenderness may be mild and localized in the upper abdomen, or it may be severe and generalized. Involuntary guarding or rigidity may not be as marked as in perforated peptic ulcer. It is unusual to find a tender mass (suggesting abscess or pseudocyst) at this stage, but the abdomen must be gently examined regularly afterwards to detect their development. Murphy's sign is positive in some cases of pancreatitis due to gall stones. Bowel sounds may be reduced or absent.

History

Reason for question	Question asked	Comment
Previous symptoms	Have you had this sort of pain before? If yes, when? On each occasion what did they say was wrong? What treatment was given?	In a patient with relapsing symptoms, think of duodenal ulcer, pancreatitis, diverticular disease, urinary tract infection or stone and cholecystitis. In such cases the patient may have experienced similar but milder pains before this episode. The absence of such 'warning' symptoms does not, however, exclude these disorders
	When were you last well and completely free of symptoms?	Before some conditions produce an intra-abdominal crisis, they may be preceded by a period of illness, weight loss and anorexia. Think especially of neoplasms in those over 50 years of age

Mode of onset of pain, its progression and characteristics	When did the pain first start? How did it start? How has it progressed since? Is it getting better or worse, or is it staying about the same? Have you been free of pain at all or is the pain continuous? When the pain comes, describe to me exactly what happens, what you do, what you take? How does the pain end? How long does the pain take to go away completely?	Record its duration in hours if less than 3 days. Avoid expressions such as 'pain started on Thursday....' Take the opportunity to decide whether this is visceral pain or colic, or whether it is due to local or general peritonitis. Pain of sudden onset (almost timed to the precise minute) occurs in perforation and acute pancreatitis. Colic occurs in small and large bowel obstruction. Think of causes in the lumen, in the wall and outside If a young woman complains of colicky pain, think of uterine or tubal origin (ectopic pregnancy or abortion). The patient often says that the pain resembles labour pain More on peritonitis below
Site of pain	Please show me where the pain is now, with one finger Show me where the pain was when it first started	As de Dombal (1991) points out, patients are more likely to give you an accurate answer if you enquire in this order *Current location in abdomen gives a useful clue to possible diagnosis:* *Right upper quadrant:* acute cholecystitis; pyelonephritis

43

Reason for question	Question asked	Comment
		Upper abdomen: perforated peptic ulcer; acute pancreatitis
		Right lower quadrant: acute appendicitis; pelvic inflammatory disease; complication of ovarian cyst
		Lower half: ectopic pregnancy; incomplete abortion; acute diverticular disease
		Left lower quadrant: acute diverticular disease; ovarian disease
		Loin: renal colic; urinary tract infection
		Generalized: perforated peptic ulcer; acute pancreatitis; leaking aortic aneurysm
		Hints from change in position of pain:
		Central pain localizing in right lower quadrant: think of appendicitis
		Upper becoming generalized: perforated peptic ulcer; acute pancreatitis
		Lower abdominal becoming generalized: perforated diverticular disease; ruptured ectopic pregnancy
		But variability of the site of the pain may well indicate non-specific abdominal pain or pain of psychogenic nature

Radiation of pain	When the pains gets worse, where does it move to? Or, where else do you feel the pain?	*Between shoulder blades from right upper quadrant:* think of acute cholecystitis; *Shoulder tip from abdomen:* ovarian cyst; ectopic pregnancy *Lumbar region of back from abdomen:* gynaecological problems; urinary tract infection; aortic aneurysm *Loin from abdomen:* renal stone; pyelonephritis *Groin or thigh from lower abdomen:* gynaecological disorder
Aggravating factors	What makes the pain worse?	Pain from local or general peritonitis is made worse by movement, coughing or sneezing. Peritonitis affecting the upper abdomen, for instance from acute cholecystitis or perforated peptic ulcer, aggravated by deep inspiration
Relieving factors	What makes the pain better? Or is there anything you can do to make the pain better?	Pain not eased by strong analgesics is severe; it occurs in general peritonitis (perforated peptic ulcer, pancreatitis, leaking aortic aneurysm). Also in renal colic Morphine makes biliary and pancreatic pain worse because it causes spasm of the sphincter of Oddi Pain from acute pancreatitis is made slightly better by sitting up and bending forward

Reason for question	Question asked	Comment
Associated features	Have you felt sick (had nausea) or have you been sick (vomited) since this pain started?	Vomiting may merely be due to severe pain, e.g. in renal colic. It may be due to gastrointestinal disease, e.g. intestinal obstruction. *As nausea and vomiting occur in a wide variety of abdominal disorders, their diagnostic value is limited. The type of vomit and the amount are useful*
	If yes, *how many times have you vomited?* *what did you bring up?* *how much of it?* *what colour was it?* *was there any blood in the vomit?*	Risk of dehydration if large volumes of fluid vomited Bile-stained vomit denotes a patent pyloric sphincter Blood in the vomit or 'coffee-ground' vomiting is due to erosions, ulceration, perforation of upper GIT. Haematemesis may also occur in acute pancreatitis. Feculent vomiting is due to severe low small bowel or large bowel obstruction
	Have you felt faint or passed out (lost consciousness)?	Fainting and loss of consciousness in a young woman suggest bleeding ectopic pregnancy

OTHER GIT SYMPTOMS (as for non-acute upper abdominal pain)		These are important for they help uncover disease that may have precipitated acute abdominal pain. Examples are: peptic ulcer leading to perforation; gall stones causing acute cholecystitis; diverticular disease that perforates Exercise care in interpreting these: the disease causing acute abdominal pain may be different from the one the patient has had for years
ROS (as for non-acute upper abdominal pain)	It is important to do a careful systems review in acute abdominal pain for several reasons: (a) to detect intercurrent disease such as diabetes, which may make an operation hazardous (b) some disorders outside the abdomen can cause acute abdominal pain, e.g. myocardial infarction; basal pneumonia (c) a history of vascular disease will be present in a proportion of patients with mesenteric ischaemia or aortic aneurysm	
PMH	**If:** Previous laparotomy Symptomatic gall stones Previous acute pancreatitis Peptic ulcer Symptomatic diverticular disease Cardiovascular disease Renal tract disease	**Think of:** Intestinal obstruction due to adhesions Acute cholecystitis Acute pancreatitis Perforated peptic ulcer Acute diverticular disease Mesenteric vascular occlusion, leaking aortic aneurysm Stone disease or infection

Reason for question	Question asked	Comment
FH	Enquire about a FH of diabetes, peptic ulcer, cancer, heart disease; appendicitis in siblings	
SH	Especially smoking and alcohol	Relevant in peptic ulcer and pancreatitis respectively
DRUGS	Steroids, aspirin, NSAIDs; anticoagulants; hypotensive and anti-diabetic agents. Antacids, ulcer healing drugs	All of these should alert you to the underlying disease for which they were prescribed. Note also drugs that cause acute pancreatitis
ALLERGIES		

EXAMINATION *General examination*	Important signs can be obtained from general examination. The patient may look ill and dehydrated from severe abdominal disorders such as perforated appendicitis, perforated peptic ulcer, severe acute pancreatitis and perforated diverticular disease. If the patient is pale and/or shocked, suspect bleeding from conditions such as ruptured ectopic pregnancy and leaking aortic aneurysm. Shock may occur from profuse vomiting from any cause, e.g. intestinal obstruction. Septic shock can be caused by perforation in any part of the gastrointestinal tract. If the patient is jaundiced, think of acute pancreatitis or cholecystitis. The temperature is often raised in local peritonitis. It may be subnormal if the patient is shocked. Fetor oris occurs in peritonitis, especially from acute appendicitis.

Age	As discussed, certain conditions are commoner at some ages: appendicitis between the ages of 10 and 30; vascular disorders such as mesenteric ischaemia and leaking aortic aneurysm in the over-70s. Do not forget the possibility of malignant disease in the elderly patient. The commonest causes of acute abdominal pain in children are mesenteric lymphadenitis, acute appendicitis, urinary tract disorders; intussusception, though uncommon, must be borne in mind.	
Sex	Do not forget gynaecological disorders in women; in women of childbearing age, complications of pregnancy (ectopic pregnancy, incomplete abortion; in young women, pelvic inflammatory disease).	
Ears, nose and throat examination	Important especially in younger patients, as upper respiratory infections may cause mesenteric lymphadenitis.	
RS	Signs of infection, collapse, consolidation, pleural effusion	Intercurrent lung and cardiovascular disease liable to complicate an operation, which may be necessary in acute abdominal pain. Also, disease above the diaphragm sometimes causes pain in the abdomen
CVS	Full cardiovascular examination noting BP, pulse, evidence of heart failure and peripheral pulses	In an elderly patient with cardiovascular signs, think of mesenteric vascular occlusion and aortic aneurysm. Atrial fibrillation should alert you to mesenteric vascular occlusion. CVS examination will help confirm the degree of shock
CNS		

49

Reason for examination	Signs looked for	Comment
ABDOMEN	Inspection: Scars	(See past medical history): previous abdominal operation predisposes to adhesions
	Discoloration	Look for Grey–Turner's sign and Cullen's sign. They are rare
	Pulsatile mass	Often transmitted pulsation, but may be an aortic aneurysm
	Does the abdomen move with respiration?	Poor movement in generalized peritonitis
	Ask patient to cough	Reluctance to cough due to severe abdominal pain seen in generalized peritonitis. If localized peritonitis present pain will occur on coughing in affected area
	Palpation: Please show me where the pain is	It is important to establish this before palpation. Be gentle and sympathetic, and avoid this area till later. de Dombal (1991) suggests leaving palpation till last
	What is the distribution of the tenderness?	This point is of the utmost importance for localizing the lesion. Sometimes the whole abdomen is tender, but it should be possible to determine the site of maximal tenderness. The whole abdomen may be equally tender. Interpretation as for 'present location of pain' in history

Is there a tender mass?	Tender mass may be appendix mass, empyema of gall bladder, twisted ovarian cyst, expanding or leaking aortic aneurysm or colonic diverticular mass. The precise location of the mass and other features such as age and sex should help you decide
Is there involuntary rigidity?	Voluntary guarding is due to fear of the examination, cold palpating hands, rough examination etc. Involuntary guarding is due to peritoneal inflammation or irritation; a useful sign if localized and the rest of the abdomen soft and non-tender
DO NOT ELICIT REBOUND TENDERNESS AT THIS STAGE.	If you hurt the patient now, he will not allow you to elicit further signs
Systematically palpate each viscus in turn.	Enlargement of or tenderness of an organ may indicate the source of the abdominal pain, as discussed above
Percussion: Tympanitic areas:	Suggest intestinal obstruction or free air in peritoneal cavity
Tenderness on light percussion:	This gives the same information as rebound tenderness
Auscultation: Increased, continuous bowel sounds	Increased and continuous bowel sounds indicate intestinal obstruction
Absent bowel sounds	Highly suggestive of peritonitis

Reason for examination	Signs looked for	Comment
	Rebound tenderness	See de Dombal (1991) for a clear description of how to elicit rebound tenderness. Correctly obtained, this sign is diagnostic of underlying peritonitis
GROINS	Hernia: reducible or irreducible? Is it tender?	May be the cause of pain or intestinal obstruction. It is imperative to exclude an external hernia in a patient with obstruction. Femoral hernias in elderly obese women are easy to miss
	Genitalia: scrotum: oedematous, inflamed. Testes: size, lie, tenderness	Pain of testicular torsion may be referred to the abdomen
RECTAL EXAMINATION	This examination and its interpretation are described in Chapter 6. In a patient with acute abdominal pain, useful points to note include masses, areas of localized tenderness and the presence of blood on the examining finger. In a patient with suspected appendicitis, for example, tenderness on the right but not the left, makes this diagnosis more likely.	
PELVIC EXAMIN- ATION IN A WOMAN	This tends to be neglected or deliberately omitted to avoid embarrassing the patient. It is evident from the list of causes of abdominal pain that gynaecological disorders are common. Every woman with abdominal pain must have pelvic examination. This must be done by the most senior member of the team in order to avoid its unnecessary repetition. Vaginal examination must be done before rectal examination.	

If:	Think of:
Mass in pelvis	Fibroids, ovarian masses, hydrosalpinx, pyosalpinx, tubo-ovarian abscess.
Tenderness, pain on moving the cervix	Tubal pregnancy, pelvic inflammatory disease.
Bleeding	Incomplete abortion
LOWER LIMBS Pulses in the lower limb	Reduced lower limb pulses may mean arterial disease elsewhere, e.g. aortic aneurysm, mesenteric arterial occlusion.

What's wrong

Important questions to be answered after history and examination include the following:

1. Is there important surgical disease? Some patients attend the accident and emergency department for reassurance. There may be no localizing features or the pain is mild and the physical findings unimpressive. It may or may not be possible to reach a firm diagnosis. It takes a lot of experience to decide that there is no serious or potentially serious disease. For instance in early acute appendicitis or if the inflamed appendix is retrocaecal, the signs may be few. If in doubt, admit. If you discharge the patient, make sure he understands which symptoms may indicate serious disease.

2. If there is disease, which organ is affected? This will be aided by the localizing features in the history and the examination.

3. What is the disease process? Is the pain colicky, is there localized peritonitis, or is there generalized peritonitis?

4. Should the diagnosis be modified in view of the patient's age and sex? The causes of intestinal obstruction are different in children from those in adults. Consider intussusception, volvulus, con-

genital lesions in children; carcinoma and diverticular disease in adults. Women with right iliac fossa peritonitis may have gynaecological disease.

5. What, if any, are the complications from this disease? For example, is the patient shocked, dehydrated or in pain? These complications need urgent treatment, as does their cause.

6. Are there any other diseases present? For instance ischaemic heart disease, chronic obstructive airways disease.

Investigations

Only the investigations normally required in the emergency period will be discussed. The investigations requested depend on the condition suspected:

Acute appendicitis

Urinalysis, Hb and WCC, U&Es may be justified if the patient has been vomiting.

Acute cholecystitis

Urinalysis, Hb, WCC, U&Es, LFTs, amylase, plain abdominal X-ray, upper abdominal ultrasound.

Acute pancreatitis

As for acute cholecystitis; serum calcium, corrected for albumin; erect X-ray of chest; supine X-ray of abdomen.

Perforated peptic ulcer

As for acute pancreatitis.

Urinary tract problem

Urinalysis, urine culture; Hb, WCC, U&Es; plain abdominal X-ray showing kidneys, ureters and bladder.

Gynaecological problem

Urinalysis, Hb, WCC, U&Es; pregnancy test in a woman of childbearing age (bearing in mind ectopic pregnancy or incomplete abortion); high vaginal swab (pelvic inflammatory disease), pelvic ultrasound.

Intestinal obstruction

Urinalysis, Hb, WCC, U&E; erect chest and supine abdominal X-ray.

Interpretation of tests in acute abdominal pain

Urine examination: Can urine be obtained? The patient may not be able to pass urine, or there may be no urine in the bladder. If the patient is seriously ill a urinary catheter should be inserted. Urine must be obtained under aseptic conditions and examined immediately. Is the urine turbid, or clear? Is it blood stained? Does it look concentrated?

Urinalysis: This should be performed in every patient with acute abdominal pain.

Specific gravity: High specific gravity urine usually due to dehydration and/or fluid deprivation.

Blood in the urine: This may be due to infection or to trauma to the urinary organs.

Protein in the urine: May be due to urinary tract infection, or to haematuria, or to a lesion in the vicinity of the bladder or ureter, for instance, an inflamed appendix.

Sugar: Glycosuria may be due to diabetes, which may be the cause of the abdominal pain, or may be an incidental finding. Glycosuria is sometimes seen in acute pancreatitis.

Bilirubin (conjugated bilirubin): This is present in urine in biliary tract obstruction. The obstruction may be intrahepatic or extrahepatic.

Urobilinogen: May be due to liver cell disease, for instance, secondary carcinoma or cirrhosis. Some urobilinogen often found in the urine in normal individuals.

Urine microscopy: This can often be done out of hours. It is indicated in some cases of suspected urinary tract infection. Pus cells and micro-organisms strengthen this diagnosis.

Hb: A low haemoglobin may be due to blood loss, e.g. from a ruptured aortic aneurysm or tubal pregnancy, or from chronic disease such as carcinoma of the stomach. It may be dietary. A normal haemoglobin does not exclude bleeding, as it may take time for the haemoglobin to drop after acute haemorrhage.

PCV or haematocrit: Often a better indicator of acute haemorrhage, as haematocrit drops before haemoglobin.

WCC: A raised white cell count may be due to dehydration or to infective or inflammatory disease. Total reliance must not be placed on the white cell count to predict inflammatory disease, for instance acute appendicitis. The white count may be normal with a gangrenous appendix, and raised with mesenteric adenitis. The higher the total white cell count, the greater the chance of acute appendicitis: in a patient suspected to have appendicitis, the likelihood of this diagnosis is 66% if the white cell count is over 15 000.

Blood urea and electrolytes: These will give an indication of the degree of dehydration and electrolyte derangement. If creatinine can be measured it will give a better idea of the extent to which raised urea is due to dehydration. Thus if the creatinine is normal and the urea raised, the uraemia is due to dehydration.

Blood sugar: Diabetes mellitus may be the cause of the abdominal pain. Hyperglycaemia also sometimes found in patients with acute pancreatitis.

Serum calcium: This must be interpreted together with the albumin. Hypercalcaemia may be the cause of abdominal pain in a patient with primary hyperparathyroidism, but such patients are unlikely to present with an acute abdomen. The calcium is often low in acute pancreatitis.

Serum amylase: A raised amylase (especially if not higher than 1500 iu/l) may be due to causes other than acute pancreatitis, for instance perforated peptic ulcer or mesenteric vascular occlusion. The amylase may be normal in acute pancreatitis if the peak has been missed in disease that has progressed for more than 24–48 hours. An amylase of more than 2000 iu/l is rarely due to a cause other than acute pancreatitis.

ECG: This may confirm atrial fibrillation in a patient suspected of having mesenteric vascular occlusion. Myocardial infarction can occasionally cause pain referred to the abdomen.

Chest X-ray: This should be done with the patient erect, and in full inspiration, if possible. It may show lung collapse, consolidation, or pleural effusion due to malignant disease or to infection. The primary neoplasm may be in the abdomen, for instance, carcinoma of the large bowel or stomach. Basal pneumonia may cause pain referred to the abdomen. Pleural effusion may be due to perforation of the oesophagus or dissection of the thoracic aorta. A widened superior mediastinum may be due to dissection of the thoracic aorta. There is a crescent of free air under the diaphragm in just over 50% of patients with perforation of a hollow intra-abdominal viscus, e.g. duodenum.

Abdominal X-rays (supine): Valuable in selected patients with acute abdominal pain. They help in diagnosing lesions such as renal and gall stones, and perforation. An X-ray of the abdomen is not necessary in certain conditions such as suspected acute appendicitis, and must be undertaken with caution in certain patients, for instance young women, who may be pregnant. The plain abdominal X-ray is valuable in diagnosing intestinal obstruction: it shows dilated loops of bowel and air–fluid levels. The erect abdominal X-ray, previously widely requested, has not been shown to add any more information to the supine film.

Ultrasound: This investigation is available in almost all modern hospitals. It is useful for diagnosing acute cholecystitis and is sometimes helpful in acute pancreatitis when bowel gas does not obscure the pancreas. In women, it is useful in detecting disorders such as ectopic pregnancy, ovarian cyst, tubo-ovarian abscess and fibroids.

Certain investigations such as IVU or other contrast X-rays are performed in emergencies. They will not be discussed further. Computers have been shown to be more accurate than doctors in diagnosing acute abdominal pain, but their use is still confined to a few centres.

Case report

Features	Analysis
Mrs Patricia Norton, a 38-year-old secretary, is married and has two young sons. She was admitted as an emergency with a 36-hour history of pain in the right upper quadrant of the abdomen and vomiting.	Note must be taken of the patient's age and sex, and also the nature of her presenting symptoms. The symptoms suggest disease in her upper abdomen, but even at this stage, disorders in the pelvis and chest must be borne in mind. However, as a student, you must think of common disorders.
Over the last 3 years, she has had mild attacks of pain in the upper abdomen, occurring about once every 6 months and lasting nearly 4 hours. As the pain has never been severe, until now, she has put it down to 'indigestion' and has taken antacids bought over the counter. The pain has never been related convincingly to food and has always subsided. Fatty foods did not seem to cause or aggravate the pain, and it did not occur at any particular time of day.	As mentioned above, in a patient with recurrent upper abdominal pain, think of diseases such as peptic ulcer, gall bladder and pancreatic disease. She is too young, and the pain is too high for diverticular disease; she may have disease in the right kidney or ureter. Do not be put off considering gall bladder disease or peptic ulcer simply because the pain is not related to food or does not wake the patient in the early hours of the morning.
On this occasion, the pain was much more severe. She had her last meal 6 hours before and had not eaten anything unusual. The pain started gradually in the right upper quadrant of the abdomen and radiated round to just below the right scapula. It was initially mild but got progressively worse over the following 5 hours until it was unbearable. At its peak, the pain was the same severity for several hours and was still in the right upper quadrant when she presented to hospital.	There may be no relation between the meal and the onset of the pain, but bear it in mind. The position and radiation of the pain are strongly in favour of gall bladder disease. This is not colicky pain; many believe that biliary pain is not colicky in the classic sense.

She felt nauseated throughout and vomited once before arriving in hospital. The vomitus comprised partially digested food and had no blood. She also felt hot and sweaty but had not fainted. She had no jaundice and her stools and urine had remained normal in colour.

Nausea and vomiting are of little diagnostic value, but as the patient vomited only once, she is unlikely to have lost much fluid and electrolytes by this means.
Her pain is probably not gynaecological but see below.
Acute cholecystitis occurs often without jaundice.

The pain was made worse by coughing, deep inspiration and movement; she preferred to lie still. She had an injection of 100 mg of pethidine i.m. after she was seen by the surgical registrar. An hour later, the pain began to get better but did not subside until 12 hours later.

Aggravation of pain by these means, and the patient's preference to lie still when the pain occurs, suggest peritonitis. Think of acute cholecystitis or pancreatitis if pain localized to the upper abdomen.

Her appetite had been good and she had gained 4 kg in the last year. There was no history of jaundice, belching of wind, abdominal pain on eating fatty foods or bloating of the abdomen. Her bowels were regular and she denied bleeding from the rectum.

Acute cholecystitis is near the top of our diagnostic probabilities, so it is important to ask about these symptoms. Absence of jaundice, belching and fatty food intolerance do not exclude this diagnosis.

There were no significant symptoms on systems review. Her periods were regular, the last one 3 weeks before this admission. She denied vaginal discharge, pain on intercourse or pain related to her periods. Micturition was normal. Other systems were normal.

In a young woman with symptoms of gall bladder disease, think of the Fitz–Hugh–Curtis syndrome and ask about gynaecological symptoms. This condition is more common than many think.

She had had no serious illnesses in the past and was not taking any regular prescribed medications.

Of course, she has been on antacids, but these were self prescribed and do not necessarily indicate that she has peptic ulcer.

Features	Analysis
On examination 2 hours after admission, she was still in pain but looked fairly well, though moderately obese. She was not anaemic or jaundiced, and was well hydrated. Temperature was 37.5°C, BP 125/75 and pulse 88/min and regular. Heart and lungs were normal apart from slight reduction in air entry at the right base of the lungs.	All these features are important in management, but do not add much to diagnosis. Again, absence of jaundice does not preclude gall bladder disease. Reduced air entry in the right base is seen in acute cholecystitis and pancreatitis, due to reduced movement of the right hemidiaphragm by upper abdominal peritonitis.
The abdomen was not distended and moved with respiration. There were no scars or discoloration. She had tenderness, muscle guarding and rigidity in the right upper quadrant. Murphy's sign was positive. The rest of the abdomen was soft and non-tender and bowel sounds were normal.	These features are highly suggestive of acute cholecystitis, but do not forget that in some patients, cholecystitis may be complicated by pancreatitis. A perforated duodenal ulcer, which has sealed, may sometimes give upper abdominal peritonitis, but not a positive Murphy's sign.

Clinical diagnosis

There are numerous features in the history and examination favouring acute cholecystitis. These are discussed at length in the text. This condition is sometimes complicated by acute pancreatitis. Much less likely are perforated peptic ulcer, right urinary tract stone and the Fitz–Hugh–Curtis syndrome; there are few symptoms and signs to support these conditions.

Investigations

Urinalysis was negative. Hb was 13.3 g/dl and WCC mildly elevated at 12.5; U&Es, LFTs, amylase were normal. The last test was repeated over several days and remained normal. Plain abdominal X-ray did not show gall stones, or free gas under the diaphragm.

Ultrasound of the upper abdomen showed a thickened gall
bladder with a 4 cm calculus. The common bile duct,
liver, pancreas and kidneys were normal. The features
were those of acute cholecystitis.

Final diagnosis
Acute calculous cholecystitis not complicated by acute pancreatitis.

References

de Dombal, F. T. (1991) *Diagnosis of Acute Abdominal
Pain* (second edition). Churchill Livingstone,
Edinburgh.
Dickson, J. A. S., Jones, A., Telfer, S. *et al.* (1988)
Scandinavian Journal of Gastroenterology, Special
Supplementum on OMGE work, **144**, 43.
Walmsley, G. L., Wilson, D. H., Gunn, A. A., Jenkins,
D., Horrocks, J. C., de Dombal, F. T. (1977) *British
Journal of Surgery*, **64**, 538.
Wilson, D. M., Wilson, P. D., Walmsley, G. *et al.* (1977)
British Journal of Surgery, **63**, 250.

Chapter 4

Surgical jaundice

Jaundice is yellow staining of the tissues due to an excess of bilirubin (conjugated or unconjugated) in the circulation. Normal bilirubin is 5–15 mmol/l, but jaundice is only detectable clinically if the bilirubin is greater than 40 mmol/l. Good natural light is needed to detect slight clinical jaundice. Tissues with a high elastic tissue content (sclera, skin) are the ones which concentrate bilirubin best.

Causes of jaundice

The causes of jaundice are *pre-hepatic, hepatic* and *post-hepatic*. In general, pre-hepatic jaundice presents to the physician and post-hepatic jaundice to the surgeon. Obstructive jaundice may be hepatic or post-hepatic. The distinction is made by ultrasound: if there is post-hepatic biliary obstruction, the bile ducts outside the liver will be dilated. Some causes of obstructive jaundice are amenable to surgical treatment.

This chapter concentrates on obstructive jaundice. Ultrasound is needed to determine whether a patient with obstructive jaundice is likely to benefit from surgical treatment.

Obstructive jaundice

The decision whether jaundice is obstructive or not can usually be made from the history: what colour are the motions and the urine? In obstructive jaundice the stools are pale and the urine dark. If in doubt, test the urine for (conjugated) bilirubin: this will be present in obstructive jaundice and absent in other types. These points are best appreciated if bilirubin metabolism is understood.

Bilirubin metabolism for the diagnostician

Bilirubin is formed from haem, a compound of iron

and protoporphyrin. There is increased production of bilirubin in disorders in which there is increased red cell breakdown, for instance administration of blood of the wrong group. This bilirubin is not soluble in water and therefore cannot be filtered into the renal tubules. It does not appear in urine and hence the jaundice which results is known as *acholuric* ('no colour in urine') jaundice.

Bilirubin is transported into the liver cell by a carrier protein. In the liver cell, bilirubin is conjugated with glucuronic acid to form bilirubin glucuronide, which is water soluble. If conjugated bilirubin 'spills' into plasma (for instance from obstruction of the bile ducts), some of it will be filtered in the kidney tubules and will appear in urine. Intrahepatic bile duct obstruction can occur from damage of liver cells in hepatitis.

Conjugated bilirubin is transported into the bile ducts and thence into the bowel. Bacteria in the bowel deconjugate bilirubin to form stercobilinogen. Some of this is reabsorbed into plasma, then taken up into the liver and recirculated (enterohepatic circulation);

some is excreted through the kidney tubules into urine as urobilinogen. It follows that if there is complete obstruction of the bile duct, there will be no urobilinogen in the urine. Also, some urobilinogen is present in the urine of the normal individual. To put this another way, if urobilinogen is present in the urine the bile duct must be patent, either partly or wholly. An increased amount of urobilinogen is present in the urine if the uptake of stercobilinogen into the liver is reduced during the enterohepatic circulation, for instance in cirrhosis of the liver.

The rest of the stercobilinogen which is not absorbed in the small bowel is passed into the colon where it is converted to stercobilin. This is the pigment which gives stools their characteristic brown colour. If stercobilin is present in excessive quantities, for instance in haemolytic disorders, faeces are dark brown in colour; if absent or reduced as in obstructive jaundice, faeces are pale or putty coloured. The table below summarizes the findings in urine and stools in the conditions commonly encountered:

	Normal	*Haemolytic disorder*	*Complete obstruction of bile ducts*	*Partial obstruction of bile ducts*	*Liver cell disease in which enterohepatic uptake reduced*
Bilirubin	0	0	+ + +	+ +	+ +
Urobilinogen	+	+ +	0	+	+ + +
Colour of stools	Normal	Dark	Pale	Normal or pale	Normal

0 = None   + = slight   + + = moderate   + + + = large

Causes of obstructive jaundice (Common causes are indicated by *)

These are (a) intrahepatic and (b) extrahepatic.

(a) Intrahepatic jaundice: (the jaundice is predominantly due to liver cell damage, hence bilirubin will be unconjugated, but there will also be intrahepatic biliary obstruction).

    Infections
        (i) Viral hepatitis*
        (ii) Infectious mononucleosis (glandular fever)
        (iii) Septicaemia*

    Poisons
        (iv) Agents such as carbon tetrachloride and aflatoxin.

    Drugs
        (v) Drugs such as halothane, tetracyclines, paracetamol and cytotoxic agents.

    Cirrhosis
        (vi) Alcohol*
        (vii) Post-hepatitic
        (viii) Cryptogenic
        (ix) Primary biliary
        (x) Cardiac failure

Tumours
   (xi) Primary carcinoma of the liver
   (xii) Secondary tumours in the liver*

(b) Extrahepatic jaundice:

   Causes within the lumen of the bile ducts
      (i) Gall stones*
   Causes in the wall of the bile ducts
      (ii) Congenital stricture and cysts
      (iii) Damage at operation
      (iv) Carcinoma of the bile duct
      (v) Carcinoma of ampulla of Vater
      (vi) Sclerosing cholangitis
   Causes outside the wall of the bile duct
      (vii) Carcinoma of the head of the pancreas*
      (viii) Acute and chronic pancreatitis*
      (ix) Enlarged lymph nodes at the porta hepatis
      (x) Other tumours, for instance carcinoma of the gall bladder.

Common causes of obstructive jaundice presenting to surgeon	Gall stones (70%), carcinoma of the head of pancreas (10%), secondary carcinoma of the liver (5%), chronic pancreatitis (5%) and acute pancreatitis (3%)

Points to look for

Certain diagnoses can be made easily from the history: for instance, paracetamol overdose causing fulminant hepatic failure. In viral hepatitis, the degree of malaise is striking compared with the jaundice, which is often transient. Secondary carcinoma of the liver is much commoner than primary hepatic carcinoma, which is very rare in western countries. Interestingly, primary hepatic neoplasms are very common in some parts of the world, for instance, China. A patient with a long history of alcohol abuse presenting with jaundice probably has cirrhosis of the liver. Cirrhosis should be suspected if there are signs of chronic liver disease, especially in the presence of portal hypertension: large spleen, oesophageal varices and ascites.

The older the patient, the more likely is jaundice to be due to malignancy.

Gall stones

Gall stone disease is common and jaundice due to stones in the common bile duct is frequently encountered. There may be a history of gall bladder disease such as upper abdominal pain. The patient characteristically presents with upper abdominal pain and jaundice which fluctuates in intensity. The gall bladder is not palpable because it is shrunken from chronic inflammation and decompresses because obstruction is incomplete and intermittent. Compare this with complete progressive obstruction from neoplasm (from Courvoisier's rule).

Courvoisier's rule (or law) states that if the gall bladder is palpable in the presence of obstructive jaundice, the jaundice is unlikely to be due to stone. The reason is that fibrosed gall bladders with stones are incapable of distending from high pressure in the obstructed biliary tree. There are exceptions to this rule. The gall bladder may not be palpable even in the presence of malignant obstruction of the common bile duct, but may be seen to be distended on ultrasound.

Carcinoma of the head of the pancreas

A tumour arising in the head of the pancreas produces obstructive jaundice by obstructing the common bile duct directly (66%), or by producing lymph nodes which obstruct the hepatic ducts at the porta hepatis (rarely). The patient may be asymptomatic until jaundice appears. The commonest symptoms are weight loss (80%), upper lumbar backache (45%) and anorexia (45%), which may be present for a long time before the jaundice appears. The jaundice is progressive and the patient will often have lost weight. A palpable gall bladder makes the diagnosis highly likely.

If the jaundice fluctuates and the gall bladder is intermittently palpable, think of periampullary carcinoma. Periampullary carcinoma can ulcerate and bleed (causing melaena), and its necrosis may lead to temporary clearance of jaundice. This is uncommon.

Secondary carcinoma of the liver

The source of the primary tumour may be obvious, for instance the patient may have been known to have carcinoma in the past; or the source of the primary tumour may be evident from the history and examination. Thus a patient presenting with jaundice who, during examination, is found to have a lump in the breast and lymph nodes in the axilla, almost certainly has a breast carcinoma with liver secondaries. It is not uncommon to have secondaries in the liver without an obvious primary tumour.

Chronic pancreatitis

The patient is often known to suffer from chronic pancreatitis. There may be a history of excessive alcohol intake. He will have had progressive lumbar backache and abdominal pain, and there may also be a history of steatorrhoea or diabetes mellitus. Patients with chronic pancreatitis are not infrequently addicted to opiate analgesics taken because of the severe pain.

Cirrhosis of the liver

This is a chronic disease affecting the whole of the liver. The liver cells are damaged and replaced by fibrous tissue and nodules of regenerating liver tissue. There are two consequences of cirrhosis by which it is diagnosed: first, there is failure of liver cell function, and second, there is portal hypertension due to obstruction to the flow of portal venous blood through the liver. There may be a causative agent such as alcohol, and a history of haematemesis and melaena due to bleeding from oesophageal varices or an associated peptic ulcer. Jaundice is seldom the only or the main presenting complaint. There will often be signs of chronic liver disease such as spider naevi, palmar erythema, and, in the male, gynaecomastia. Signs of portal hypertension (see above) may be present.

History

Reason for question	Question asked	Comment
Find out about duration and progression of jaundice	When was jaundice or yellowness first discovered? Where was the yellowness most apparent, in the eyes or on the skin?	Jaundice appearing within a week is common in hepatitis, which may be due to drugs, toxins, viruses or bacteria. Jaundice over the course of weeks is typical of extrahepatic biliary obstruction whether due to tumour, pancreatitis or stricture of the common bile duct

Reason for question	Question asked	Comment
	How has the jaundice progressed? Has it progressively deepened, has it got lighter or is it fluctuating?	Progressive jaundice is common in carcinoma. Jaundice which appears and then fades rapidly may be due to hepatitis or to a toxic agent
		Fluctuating jaundice is due to gall stones in most cases but occasionally it is due to a tumour, especially periampullary carcinoma
Any recent illness or constitutional symptoms?	How have you felt in yourself before and during the course of the jaundice? Have you been unwell?	Anorexia, nausea and vomiting, especially associated with weight loss within 2 weeks of the appearance of jaundice, suggests hepatitis or biliary obstruction secondary to gall stones. If these symptoms appear for more than 2 weeks before the appearance of jaundice, the cause is more likely to be a toxin, especially alcohol. Patients with malignant obstruction are usually well before they become jaundiced
	Has your weight changed recently? By how much and over how long?	Profound weight loss with jaundice should suggest malignancy, but it is seen in the early stages of viral hepatitis

Any accompanying features?	Have you had any itching?	Itching is due to accumulation of bile salts in the tissues in obstructive jaundice, and may be noticed many days before jaundice is apparent. Pruritus of a few weeks is common in large duct obstruction due to neoplasm or intrahepatic cholestasis from drugs. If present for several months or years in a middle-aged woman, pruritus suggests primary biliary cirrhosis
	Have you had fever or shivering attacks?	Fever is due to acute cholecystitis or to cholangitis following obstruction of the common bile duct by stone
	Have you had pain anywhere? If so determine its location and characteristics as described earlier	This is an important symptom and is most valuable when volunteered by the patient
Is the pain typical of gall bladder disease?	See earlier notes	Pain should suggest gall stones, but is occasionally absent. Painless obstructive jaundice is typical of carcinoma of the biliary tract or head of the pancreas. A history of lumbar backache suggests chronic pancreatitis or carcinoma of the pancreas

Reason for question	*Question asked*	*Comment*
Any predisposing cause?	Do you belch wind or burp a lot? Do fatty foods upset you? If yes, in what way? Do you suffer from bloating of your tummy?	These symptoms suggest chronic gall bladder disease
	Have you had any blood transfusions or injections? If yes describe circumstances	Risk of infective hepatitis. Addicts often do not admit drug abuse
ROS	Finish GIT enquiry	The liver is a common site for secondaries from malignancies of most organs, especially the GI tract
	History of haematemesis and melaena?	Cirrhosis of the liver causes portal hypertension and oesophageal varices. Bleeding may be from varices or from gastritis or associated duodenal ulcer
	RS:	Consider primary carcinoma of the respiratory tract or secondaries from another organ affecting the liver and the lungs
	CVS:	Congestive cardiac failure can cause jaundice
	CNS: Ask close relative about the patient's behaviour, memory and intellect	Think of secondaries in the brain. Look for evidence of hepatic encephalopathy
	GUS: Any signs of gynaecological cancer in women, and of urinary cancer in both sexes?	

PMH	Any previous or recent operations? Were blood transfusions given during these operations?	Especially operations performed for cancer or gall stones. In patients who have had multiple operations, think of halothane as a cause of jaundice. In a patient who has had a biliary operation, think of injury to or stones retained in the common bile duct
FH	Family history of gall stones and cancer	
SH	Alcohol: document exact intake	Excessive ingestion points to cirrhosis or chronic pancreatitis
	Drug abuse	Risk of infective hepatitis
	Country of origin	Primary carcinoma of the liver commoner in people from southern Africa and the Far East
DRUGS	Use of hepatotoxic drugs and general anaesthetic agents Exposure to toxic agents	Drugs that damage the liver include paracetamol, aspirin, oral contraceptives, anabolic steroids and tetracycline Halothane, used widely in anaesthesia, rarely produces hepatitis in patients repeatedly exposed to it
ALLERGIES		

Examination

Reason for examination	Sign elicited	Comment
General well-being, state of nutrition, depth of jaundice	Think of carcinoma of the pancreas or chronic pancreatitis in a patient who is unwell, thin and anaemic and has jaundice.	
	Any skin scratch marks?	Pruritus common in obstructive jaundice
	Purpura	Due to clotting derangement
	Oedema	Due to malnutrition (low plasma proteins), heart or liver failure
	Lymphadenopathy, especially enlarged supraclavicular nodes	Consider carcinoma of the pancreas
	Raised temperature	If intermittent, suggests cholangitis, more common in gall stone disease
Signs of hepatic encephalopathy and examination of the rest of CNS	Fetor hepaticus Flapping tremor Confused, altered mood or behaviour Speech inarticulate Drowsy; inappropriate behaviour Able to obey only simple commands Comatose, responding only to pain	Increasing severity of hepatic encephalopathy
	Tendon reflexes	Reflexes are exaggerated in the early stages, but disappear in the late stages

Signs of chronic liver disease	Spider naevi Palmar erythema Finger clubbing	
	Gynaecomastia and testicular atrophy in males	Due to failure by liver to degrade circulating oestrogens
RS	Any signs of lung collapse, consolidation or effusion?	These may be due to secondary carcinoma
CVS		
ABDOMEN *Abdominal examination most important in obstructive jaundice*	*Inspection:* Any scars?	From previous operations, especially for cancer or gall stones
	Distension?	Is distension due to a large tumour, enlarged liver or to ascites?
	Any dilated veins?	Due to portal venous obstruction
	Palpation: Tenderness, especially in the right upper quadrant?	Due to an enlarged liver in viral hepatitis or tender gall bladder
	Examine the liver: Is it palpable? What is its size and consistency? Its edge? Is it nodular, any large nodules palpable in it?	Enlarged nodular liver or liver with discrete nodules in carcinoma
		Firm liver edge in cirrhosis. In late stage cirrhosis the liver is small

Reason for examination	Sign elicited	Comment
	Is gall bladder palpable?	If gall bladder palpable, obstructive jaundice is more likely to have been caused by malignant obstruction than by stones (Courvoisier's law – Mann and Russell, 1992)
	Is the spleen palpable? What is its size?	Enlarged spleen indicates portal hypertension, most commonly due to cirrhosis of the liver
	Any other abnormal masses?	Suggesting malignancy, for instance of the stomach or colon
	Percussion: Shifting dullness	Examine for ascites
	Auscultation	
	Rectal examination: any masses, blood or mucus?	Think of rectal carcinoma
	In the male, is the prostate normal or does it feel irregular?	Consider prostatic carcinoma
	Vaginal examination in a woman: examine vulva, vagina, cervix, uterus and ovaries; any abnormalities of these organs?	Do not forget cancer of the genital organs

Investigations

All patients presenting with jaundice should have the following investigations:

Urine examination: Look at the urine. It will be dark and frothy. Test it for bilirubin and urobilinogen. Bilirubin is present in obstructive jaundice. Note that some urobilinogen is present even in normal individuals. Excessive amounts of urobilinogen suggest its defective uptake by the liver in the enterohepatic circulation, and occurs in cirrhosis of the liver. Urobilinogen is absent if the obstruction is complete.

Examination of the stool: Look at the stool. It is pale or putty coloured in obstructive jaundice.

Hb, WCC, platelets: Anaemia may occur in carcinoma and in chronic pancreatitis.

ESR or CRP: This may be raised in a patient with malignancy or infective hepatitis.

Clotting screening: Clotting tests are abnormal in obstructive jaundice because of the failure to absorb vitamin K. Also, prothrombin synthesis is reduced in hepatic disease. These tests should be done before the patient is started on vitamin K. Do them early if invasive tests such as percutaneous cholangiogram and operation are contemplated.

Urea and electrolytes: These are useful if ascites is present. The accumulation of fluid in the peritoneal cavity can cause electrolyte imbalance.

LFTs: These are of great value. Do bilirubin (conjugated and unconjugated if necessary), alkaline phosphatase, albumin, globulin, transaminase, gamma glutamyl transpeptidase. The level of bilirubin reflects the degree of obstruction.

Immunological tests: Hepatitis B surface antigen test must be done in all jaundiced patients. If carcinoma suspected, do alpha-1 fetoprotein, which may be raised in hepatocellular carcinoma. Carcinoembryonic antigen (CEA) may be a useful marker for gut tumours.

Chest X-ray: This may show secondary carcinoma in the lungs or mediastinal lymph nodes.

Plain X-ray of the abdomen: Look for radio-opaque gall stones, pancreatic calcification (chronic pancreatitis), and ground-glass appearance suggesting ascites.

Ultrasound scan of the upper abdomen: This should be done within 48 hours of the patient arriving in the hospital. It is valuable because it is non-invasive and gives useful information. The following areas can be examined:

The *peritoneal cavity* for ascites.
The *liver* for size, architecture, focal defects indicating carcinoma (primary or secondary). Dilated intrahepatic ducts are diagnostic of 'surgical' jaundice.
Porta hepatis for lymph nodes.
Extra-hepatic ducts for size, filling defects such as gall stones and tumours. Tumours difficult to diagnose unless very large. An important rule to bear in mind is that dilated extra-hepatic ducts are diagnostic of post-hepatic obstruction.
Gall bladder for size, contents (gall stones, sludge), thickness (chronic inflammation) and tumour within it.
Pancreas for size, texture, tumours, pancreatic duct size. The pancreas is not infrequently obscured by overlying bowel gas.

Portal vein for size. This is important if cirrhosis is suspected.
Spleen for size (in portal hypertension).
Para-aortic area for lymph nodes which may be due to lymphoma or secondary carcinoma.

Also do ultrasound of the lower abdomen if pelvic disease such as ovarian tumour suspected.

Study the results of the above to determine whether further investigations are indicated. Thus, if the patient has multiple secondaries in the liver, there may be no indication for further investigations unless this diagnosis is in doubt. One must always question the need to look for the source of obscure primary lesions when there are multiple secondaries; occasionally, of course, such a search is justified, for instance if lymphoma is suspected.

Further investigations

Barium meal: This may show a carcinoma in the oesophagus or stomach. Carcinoma of the head of the pancreas widens the loop of the duodenum; often this tumour is extensive and advanced.

Upper GIT endoscopy: Will enable biopsies to be taken of suspicious lesions. It is particularly useful if a periampullary carcinoma of the duodenum is present for this lesion can be inspected and biopsied.

Needle biopsy of the liver: Coagulation defects must first be corrected. It is useful if a primary hepatocellular carcinoma and cirrhosis of the liver are suspected. Sometimes it is important to obtain histological proof of carcinoma, especially if ultrasound scan is equivocal. In the presence of obstructive jaundice, liver biopsy can cause severe bleeding.

Percutaneous transhepatic cholangiography (PTC): In this technique, a fine needle is introduced into the liver through the skin of the right lower chest wall. The needle is aspirated constantly until bile can be drawn freely. Radiographic contrast is injected to outline the intra- and extra-hepatic biliary ducts. The test is done after correction of coagulation defects, and is indicated in a patient with extrahepatic biliary obstruction in whom an operation would be considered. It will show the site and nature of the obstruction (benign or malignant stricture), and the anatomy of the biliary tree above the obstruction.

Endoscopic retrograde cholangio-pancreatography (ERCP): In this investigation, a long fibreoptic endoscope is passed into the duodenum and the duodenal papilla found and cannulated. Contrast is injected to outline the pancreatic and biliary ducts. It is indicated in chronic pancreatitis, in carcinoma of the biliary and pancreatic ducts (to supplement information gained from PTC, rarely), and sometimes in the investigation of obstruction by gall stones. It will demonstrate gall stones in the common duct, strictures of the bile ducts, abnormalities such as strictures and stones in the pancreatic duct suggesting chronic pancreatitis and evidence of pancreatic tumours. ERCP can also be combined with techniques for obtaining cytological specimens from the pancreatic ducts, for the removal of stones in the common bile duct, and for introducing catheters through strictures in the common bile duct. A stent can also be inserted through a malignant stricture of the lower bile duct.

CT scanning of the abdomen: This is an expensive investigation and is indicated if carcinoma of the pancreas is suspected. It may show tumours in all parts of the pancreas. It will often also show dilated pancreatic ducts.

Coeliac and superior mesenteric artery angiograms: These demonstrate the anatomy of these vessels and their branches, and are useful to show aberrations in the anatomy of these branches. Thus the hepatic artery often comes off the superior mesenteric artery rather than the coeliac axis, and would be damaged in the course of an operation if the anatomy was not known. This test is used only when the lesion has been diagnosed and surgery is being planned. Occasionally, it may show small tumours of the pancreas.

The last three tests, namely PTC, CT scanning and angiography, are best carried out on specialist hepato-biliary units where complex operations are carried out on the liver, bile ducts and pancreas. They are invasive and expensive.

It should be pointed out that the diagnosis of carcinoma of the pancreas is still crude and inaccurate. Tumours can be missed even by the above tests.

Case report

Features	Analysis
Mr Tom Jackson, a retired solicitor, is aged 69. He lives in the country with his wife, a retired nurse. His illness started at least 6 months before when they went to stay with their daughter; she noticed that his eyes were yellow.	It is not uncommon for jaundice to be discovered by someone other than the patient when there are no other symptoms. Consider causes such as hepatitis, cirrhosis of the liver and of course at this age, malignancy. Gall stones usually present with pain but cannot be ruled out.
He was well in himself and had not had any recent illnesses. His appetite was good and his weight steady. His stools were pale and his urine dark, but he had no itching. He had no pain in his abdomen. He saw his daughter's GP	This man had developed painless obstructive jaundice without antecedent illness. This is unusual in most forms of viral hepatitis, where there is often malaise, anorexia and other symptoms of infection, but these may be mild

who suggested that the patient saw his own GP as soon as he returned home. The jaundice got more pronounced over the next week, the urine got darker and the stools paler. However, the patient remained fairly well in himself and by the time he was home 2 weeks later, the jaundice practically cleared and the stools and urine returned to normal. He did not see his GP as instructed because he felt well.

Five months later, he developed jaundice again and the urine was dark and the stools pale, as earlier. On this occasion, however, he developed anorexia and lost 5 kg in 4 weeks. He had no pain, fever or rigors. The jaundice became deeper, so he consulted his GP who referred him to hospital.

On questioning, he admitted to having passed black stools for 2 days while he was at his daughter's house, but this had cleared. His bowels were regular.

There were no significant symptoms on review of systems. He was not on regular medication. He had not been abroad in the last 15 years and had had no blood transfusions or injections. He was a non-smoker but had drunk 24 units of alcohol (mainly whisky) for over 40 years.

or so far from the jaundice that the patient may not appreciate the association.

Jaundice which clears only to recur should raise the possibility of gall stones but the absence of pain makes this diagnosis less likely. Jaundice due to malignancy usually progressive but may fluctuate in periampullary carcinoma. The association with anorexia and weight loss should alert us to the possibility of malignancy.

This suggests upper GIT bleeding if the patient has not been on drugs such as iron, which make stools dark. Upper GIT bleeding in the presence of jaundice should make you think of oesophageal varices due to cirrhosis of the liver; or peptic ulcers and gastric erosions, which are a common source of bleeding in patients with cirrhosis. Necrosis of periampullary tumour rarely causes melaena.

Drug-induced jaundice must always be borne in mind, as should hepatitis B. The level of this man's alcohol intake puts him at risk of cirrhosis.

Features	Analysis
He looked well though obviously jaundiced. There were no signs of chronic liver disease such as spider naevi or palmar erythema. There were no enlarged lymph nodes. BP was 150/90 and pulse 80/min and regular. Heart and lungs were normal.	The absence of stigmata of chronic liver disease does not rule out cirrhosis.
The abdomen was not distended and there were no dilated veins. On palpation, the abdomen was soft and non-tender. The liver was enlarged 2 cm below the right costal margin and in the right hypochondrium was a 3 cm smooth mass that moved down with inspiration. The spleen was not palpable and there was no ascites.	Hepatomegaly may be due to biliary obstruction or tumour. The mass in the right hypochondrium may be a distended gall bladder, suggesting malignancy obstructing the common bile duct (from Courvoisier's rule). It may be a tumour in the liver (primary or secondary), or a tumour of the gall bladder (infiltrating the common duct and causing obstructive jaundice).
His genitalia were normal. Rectal examination showed a slightly enlarged, smooth prostate and pale stools, but no masses. All peripheral pulses were normal.	This is objective confirmation that the stools are pale.

Clinical diagnosis
The features are so typical of periampullary carcinoma that the diagnosis can often be made from the history alone. In favour of this diagnosis are his age, the insidious onset and intermittent nature of the jaundice, the absence of pain and the occurrence of melaena followed by improvement of jaundice. However, bear in mind gall stones and cirrhosis of the liver, but they are less likely.

Investigations

There was a large amount of bilirubin and no urobilinogen in the urine. Hb and U&Es were normal. Bilirubin was 955 μmol/l (normal < 22), alanine aminotransferase (ALT) 250 U/l (5–40), gamma glutamyl transpeptidase (γGT) 650 U/l (11–51) and alkaline phosphatase 1550 U/l (70–330).

This suggests complete biliary obstruction.

Raised bilirubin and alkaline phosphatase are diagnostic of biliary obstruction. Liver cell damage, resulting in raised ALT, is seen in longstanding biliary obstruction; this man's alcohol intake is a strong factor. This is even more likely in view of the raised γGT.

Prothrombin time was prolonged.

This is due to the combination of biliary obstruction and liver cell damage.

Hepatitis B surface antigen was negative.

This is an important test. Hepatitis B must be considered in all jaundiced patients.

Ultrasound of the abdomen showed a slightly enlarged liver with dilated intrahepatic ducts but no secondaries. The common bile duct was dilated and the gall bladder grossly distended, but there were no stones. The pancreas was obscured by gas but did not appear to have a mass.

Dilatation of the bile ducts confirms obstruction. In this patient the level is the lower common bile duct or pancreas.

Ultrasound can miss small tumours in the head of the pancreas, the common bile duct and the periampullary region.

ERCP showed a polypoid, ulcerated tumour on the left wall of the duodenum, at the level of the papilla. Biopsies were taken.

These are the features of a periampullary carcinoma.

Chest X-ray was normal.

Think of the possibility of lung secondaries.

81

Final diagnosis
Periampullary carcinoma. Mild cirrhosis of the liver.

Reference

Mann, C. V., Russell, R. C. G. (editors) (1992) *Bailey & Love's Short Practice of Surgery* (21st edition). Chapman & Hall Medical, London, p. 1069.

Chapter 5

Acute upper gastrointestinal bleeding

This manifests as haematemesis and/or melaena. Haematemesis should be distinguished from haemoptysis. The causes can be classified into local and systemic disorders. The amount of blood lost cannot be judged from the amount vomited. Also, melaena is not a good indication of current bleeding—the blood being passed per rectum may have been shed many hours or even days beforehand. Upper gastrointestinal bleeding is a potentially serious condition. An important condition to recognize early is oesophageal varices, for its treatment requires special skills.

The aim of this chapter is to illustrate the ways in which emergency treatment is integrated into history and examination. It emphasizes treatment of the potentially life-threatening condition, while at the same time encouraging the student to obtain a full history and do a full examination if possible. The specific treatment of the different causes of haematemesis is not discussed.

Causes of haematemesis and melaena (those which commonly cause life-threatening bleeding are marked *)

These can be classified into (a) local and (b) systemic causes.

(a) Local causes:
   (i) Diseases of the oesophagus
      –Reflux oesophagitis
      –Oesophageal varices*
   (ii) Diseases of the stomach
      –Gastritis* for instance from drugs such as aspirin, NSAIDS
      –Gastric ulcer*
      –Gastric carcinoma
      –Mallory–Weiss syndrome
   (iii) Diseases of the duodenum
      –Ulcer*
      –Erosions

(b) Systemic causes:
   (i) Anticoagulant treatment
   (ii) Other bleeding and clotting disorders

Common causes of acute upper gastrointestinal bleeding

Duodenal ulcer (40%), gastric ulcer (20%). Other common causes are gastric and duodenal erosions (together 25%) and oesophagitis (5%).

Less common but important causes

Oesophageal varices (2%), carcinoma of the stomach (1%) and Mallory–Weiss tears (1%).

Points to look for

The onset and progression of the bleeding do not give an indication of the cause, merely of its severity. However, a good history will in many cases enable a diagnosis to be made of the underlying cause of bleeding. The patient may have been diagnosed to suffer from one of the above conditions, but bleeding may not be due to the condition. About 10% of patients with oesophageal varices presenting with upper gastrointestinal haemorrhage are bleeding from gastritis or a duodenal ulcer.

Gastritis

History of recurrent upper abdominal, nausea and vomiting. Patient may be known to be taking drugs such as NSAIDs and indeed the acute episode of upper gastrointestinal bleeding may follow ingestion of this drug. Or it may follow an excessive intake of alcohol.

Some NSAIDs have been reported to cause upper GI bleeding more often than others. The drug azapropazone is reported to cause bleeding most frequently, followed by piroxicam and ketoprofen. Lower frequencies were reported with diclofenac, naproxen and indomethacin; lowest with ibuprofen. During the history, it is important to identify the drugs the patient has been taking.

Duodenal ulcer

There is often a long history to suggest duodenal ulcer (Chapter 3).

Oesophagitis

Discussed in Chapters 1 and 2.

Oesophageal varices

Past history of cirrhosis of the liver in 40%.
Previous diagnosis and treatment of oesophageal varices in 10%.
Signs of chronic liver disease such as spider naevi and palmar erythema in 10%.
Enlarged spleen and ascites in 90%.

Immediate management

Assess rapidly

How much blood has been lost and over how long? The amount of blood actually seen by the patient is not a good guide to the amount lost. There is more blood in the gut than is shed either through vomiting or as melaena or both. On the other hand, even a small amount of blood may seem a lot to the patient. Assessment must be based on clinical features. They depend on three factors taken together:

(a) The amount of blood lost;
(b) The time over which it is lost, i.e. the speed with which the patient bleeds;
(c) The response of the patient to the blood lost. This depends to some extent on the patient's cardiovascular system. A patient with cardiovascular disease becomes shocked much earlier and more profoundly than one with a previously normal cardiovascular system for the same amount of blood loss.

The following is a rough guide and applies to adults with previously normal haemoglobin levels (Bailey, 1988). It is important to note that a loss of even 500 ml over a few minutes may result in hypotension in some.

Note severity of bleeding

Category 1

Loss of less than 800 ml of blood over about 3 or 4 hours: the patient looks reasonably well and is orientated. He looks pink, his systolic BP is 120 mmHg or more and his pulse less than 90/min. The volume of the pulse is usually normal. If a central venous pressure (CVP) line is inserted, the CVP will be greater than 6 cm of water. If his urine output is measured over the next hour it is over 40 ml.

Category 2

Loss of 1–2 litres of blood over about 4 hours: the patient is restless and pale and has a cold periphery. Systolic BP is between 90 and 100 mmHg with the patient lying flat and pulse rate between 90 and 100/min. If the systolic blood pressure is taken with the patient sitting up, there is a postural drop of less than 10 mmHg. The volume of the pulse is reduced but it is not thready. If a CVP line is inserted the pressure will be between 0 and 5 cm of water, and urine volume over the next hour will be less than 25 ml. If he is given 500 ml of blood over the next 30 minutes, his systolic BP will rise to about 110 mmHg but will fall back to the original level within 30 minutes of the transfusion.

Category 3

Loss of over 2.5 litres: the patient is anxious and confused. He is cold, clammy and pale. Breathing is fast, deep and laboured. Systolic BP is less than 75 mmHg and the pulse rate is over 130 and the volume is thready. There is a postural drop of blood pressure of more than 10 mmHg. CVP is less than minus 5 cm water and there will no urine output over the next hour. His blood pressure will not respond to a transfusion of 500 ml of blood over 30 minutes.

It may take at least an hour or two before the true category in which a patient falls is established, but current decisions can be made from the patient's condition, blood pressure and pulse.

Set up an IV line or lines

For patients in category 1, one good IV line (e.g. a grey Venflon) is enough. For the others, two good lines must be established. If the patient is collapsed and it is difficult to get a satisfactory drip, a line is inserted into the internal jugular or subclavian vein. CVP measurement is important because clinical monitoring alone of the patient's progress is unreliable.

Take blood samples

Blood is taken from the IV cannula before the infusion is started. Send for Hb, WCC, PCV, platelets; U&Es and clotting studies for all patients. Group and save serum for category 1 patients, and cross match 4 units for category 2, and 6 units for category 3. If in doubt about the true category, cross match 2 units.

If oesophageal varices suspected, for instance because of past history of cirrhosis, also send blood to the laboratory for the following: LFTs, hepatitis B surface antigen and prothrombin time. These assays should be performed immediately.

What fluid?

The best fluid to replace blood is, of course, whole blood but the crucial treatment at this stage is to replace circulating volume, which is more important than replacing red cells. If plasma expanders (colloids) are available, for instance human plasma protein fraction, haemaccel, dextran 70, hetastarch, they should be given. If not, give crystalloids such as dextrose, dextrose saline or normal saline. Whatever fluid is available must be given in adequate volume.

Precautions

If you give dextrose, make sure that the line is flushed with normal saline before blood is given through it, because dextrose is liable to cause the blood to clot in the line.

Some fluids, notably dextran, interfere with blood cross matching. If such a fluid is to be used, enough blood must be obtained first for cross matching.

The place of unmatched O Rhesus negative blood

It may take 30 minutes, and in some cases considerably longer, for cross matched blood to be available. Patients in categories 1 and 2 who are responding to colloids or crystalloids can usually wait for matched blood. Those in category 3 not responding must be given blood; unmatched O Rh negative blood is used if the risk of a transfusion reaction in such a case is judged to be less than that of death from continuing haemorrhage.

How much and how fast

Do not wait for the haemoglobin result if the clinical

features indicate that significant blood loss has occurred or is occurring. In any case, in acute blood loss, a single Hb level is a poor guide to the volume of blood lost. If category 1, give 500 ml of blood or other fluid over 30 minutes and measure response (BP, pulse rate and the volume of the pulse). Reduce infusion rate to say 500 ml in 1 hour if BP sustained and the pulse volume increased.

If category 2 or 3, give the first 1000 ml of fluid as quickly as it will go, in 5–10 minutes if necessary. Check response; if no change in BP and pulse, continue giving fluid at this rate until the BP rises and the pulse volume increases. Pulse may take time to fall. Watch the JVP and listen to the lung bases for fine crackles. If JVP rises to up to 5 cm or crackles appear, slow the transfusion to 500 ml every 1 hour and monitor progress. It may be necessary to speed up the transfusion or to reduce it depending on further pro-gress. The aim in acute gastrointestinal haemorrhage is to restore the circulating volume to normal or near normal, for if the patient should start bleeding again, he has a greater chance of survival if his blood volume is close to ideal.

Do not raise the systolic BP to a level greater than 120 mmHg and the CVP (if used) to above 5 cm water, otherwise clot formation and retraction at the bleed-ing site will be discouraged and bleeding will continue.

Further management and monitoring

Explain to patient what you are doing and reassure him.
Continue monitoring.

When condition stable, proceed to full history and examination.

History

Reason for question	Question asked	Comment
Was it blood, and if so was it coughed or vomited?	Please tell me what the problem is You say you have brought up blood. What makes you think it was blood. Describe it to me Where did the blood come from?	Allow the patient to describe his symptoms. It seems almost unnecessary to ask these questions, but a lot of time and effort will be saved if it is established that what the patient has brought up is blood and not, for example, red wine. Avoid words like 'coffee-grounds', which may mislead
The form and severity of the blood loss. Health immediately before bleeding	Have you vomited blood before? How have you been in yourself in the last few days or weeks? Did you have any warning that you were going to vomit blood? How did the bleeding start?	Previous history of bleeding, e.g. from DU. About a third of patients with peptic ulcers do not have symptoms before they bleed. Almost half of the patients who bleed have no symptoms to suggest the cause of the bleeding
	How much have you vomited? (Describe in cupfuls, pints, etc.)	The patient is better able to describe volume of blood lost in familiar measures, rather than in millilitres. Remember however that even a little blood seems a lot to a frightened patient or relatives. There is almost always more blood lost than appears in vomit
Rectal blood loss	What has the colour of your motions been? Please describe your motions How much of these motions have you been passing?	Blood in the rectum in a patient with haematemesis indicates severe bleeding

Reason for question	Question asked	Comment
Symptoms accompanying blood loss	How have you felt since you started vomiting blood?	These may give an indication of the severity of blood loss
	Have you felt giddy or light-headed?	
	Have you felt your heart thumping inside your chest? (palpitations)	
	Have you felt any pain in your chest? (describe)	Angina and palpitations may accompany severe anaemia
Possible cause of bleeding Drugs	What tablets have you been taking, how much and for how long?	These drugs cause gastric erosions
	Ask about tablets for backache or headaches (aspirin), tablets for arthritis (phenylbutazone, indomethacin); and steroids	
	Do you take blood-thinning tablets (anticoagulants)?	
Benign upper GIT lesion	Any history of indigestion, heartburn, or pain in the upper part of your tummy? Do you wake up in the middle of the night with tummy pain?	Peptic ulcer, reflux oesophagitis, hiatus hernia
Malignancy	What has your appetite been like?	Carcinoma of stomach a rare cause of haematemesis (see above)
	Enquire about weight loss. If yes, how much and over how long?	

Cirrhosis of liver	How much alcohol do you drink? How long have you been drinking? Have you ever had diseases such as cirrhosis of your liver, or hepatitis?	Cirrhosis of the liver presents with upper GIT bleeding in 25% of patients known to have this liver disorder
ROS	*Rest of GIT*: RS, *CVS*, CNS, GUS	Think of intercurrent disease, which will have to be taken into account in management. An example is ischaemic heart disease
PMH	DU, gastric ulcer, cirrhosis of the liver, hepatitis Arthritis, chronic pain requiring analgesics Recent major operation Deep venous thrombosis or pulmonary embolism	Suggests stress ulceration Requiring anticoagulant treatment
DRUGS	As mentioned earlier, aspirin, steroids, other NSAIDS, anticoagulants	
FH	Family history of peptic ulcer, bleeding disorders, liver disease	
SH	Alcohol intake: document type of drinks, quantities in an average week, how long the patient has been drinking (covered above) Does he 'binge' drink?	Do not forget cirrhosis of the liver
	Drug abuse Smoking	Risk of hepatitis Increased risk of peptic ulcer
ALLERGIES		

Examination

Reason for examination	Sign elicited	Comment
General examination	Take time now to assess the patient more thoroughly. He may look ill from an underlying disease such as malignancy or simply from blood loss. He may be anaemic and dehydrated from bleeding. Enlarged lymph nodes should alert you to the possibility of malignancy. Bruising and purpura suggest platelet deficiency	
General signs of chronic liver disease	Spider naevi, palmar erythema, gynaecomastia, clubbing of the fingers, testicular atrophy in males	
Signs of liver failure	Jaundice, fetor hepaticus, flapping tremor, confusion	
RS	Signs of collapse, consolidation, pleural effusion, infection	These may be due to secondary tumours in the lungs
CVS	BP, pulse, JVP, apex beat, thrills, murmurs, added sounds	As indicated above, they aid in the assessment of the degree of shock and in determining whether the patient is in heart failure.
CNS	Confused (as above)	May be because of shock or liver failure
	Focal neurological deficit	This suggests secondaries in brain
	Generalized impairment such as increased tone, reflexes, poor coordination	This is more in keeping with neurological impairment due to hepatic failure

ABDOMEN	*Inspection:* Scars from previous operations	e.g. for peptic ulcer, varices, carcinoma
	Distension	May be due to ascites from liver failure or secondary carcinoma
	Visible masses	May be enlarged liver, spleen or tumour deposit
	Abnormal veins	Think of portal hypertension
	Palpation: Enlarged liver	Consider portal hypertension and liver secondaries
	Enlarged spleen	portal hypertension
	Abnormal masses	tumour deposits
	Tenderness	Epigastric tenderness suggests peptic ulcer
	Percussion: Shifting dullness	To detect ascites
	Auscultation:	
	PR: melaena, blood	The presence of blood or melaena supports the history of bleeding. Black tarry stools may be due to oral iron
	Masses felt on rectal examination	Think of pelvic secondaries from carcinoma of stomach

Further investigations

Upper GIT endoscopy: This must be carried out as soon as feasible, for it enables a diagnosis to be made early in the course of the bleeding and operation planned when it is most appropriate. Another important role of endoscopy is in therapy. For example, varices can be injected at the time of endoscopy.

Barium meal: This is difficult to interpret because of the large quantity of blood and clots in the stomach and duodenum. It is of greater value in investigating the cause of bleeding when the bleeding has stopped.

Case report

Features	Analysis
Mr Jack Wilson is aged 37. He is a painter and decorator, and is married with two children. He presented to the accident and emergency department with a 4-hour history of vomiting blood.	Note the patient's age and sex. Benign conditions such as peptic ulcer more common than malignancies. Younger patients tolerate acute bleeding more than the elderly.
He had never vomited blood before. He was well before this episode but came home in the evening complaining of lightheadedness and feeling unwell and had to lie down. Half an hour later, he started retching and, shortly after, he vomited a mixture of fresh and dark blood, with clots. He said he vomited 3 cupfuls by the time the ambulance called by his wife arrived. During the 15-minute journey, he vomited another 2 cupfuls. He had last opened his bowels the previous day and not noticed any blood in the stool. The stool colour was normal.	Two-thirds of patients presenting with bleeding feel unwell and have symptoms in the hour or two before they vomit. A cupful is about 300 ml. It is estimated that the patient vomited 1500 ml of blood, but this is a rough estimate.

For the past 2 years he had had intermittent bouts of upper abdominal pain, sometimes waking him up in the early hours of the morning. He took antacids and cimetidine tablets bought directly over the counter. As these medicines have always cleared the pain, he had ignored advice from his chemist to consult his GP.

The history suggests peptic ulcer. This may well be the cause of bleeding, but in nearly a third of patients presenting with haematemesis, there are two lesions present, and only one is the source of haemorrhage.

His appetite was good and his weight steady and he denied jaundice. His bowels were regular.

Always think of all possible causes of bleeding, including malignancy and oesophageal varices.

He had no other symptoms on systems review and had had no significant illnesses or operations in the past. He drank 18 units of alcohol a week and had smoked 25 cigarettes a day for 20 years.

Absence of intercurrent illness is an advantage for the patient, but chest infection and hypoxia are likely if an operation is performed. 18 units of alcohol are considered 'safe' but true intake may be more than the patient admits to. Smoking is an important risk factor for peptic ulcer.

On examination he was pale, sweaty and anxious, but otherwise looked reasonably well and did not appear shocked. He was not jaundiced and had no signs of liver disease.

Always think of oesophageal varices due to cirrhosis of the liver among the causes of upper GI haemorrhage.

BP was 105/70 on lying down and 100/65 on sitting up. Pulse was 96/min, regular and of good volume. Heart and lungs were normal and all peripheral pulses were present and normal.

A postural drop of 5 mmHg, together with history and features on examination, suggests blood loss of Category 2 above, but this is approximate.

Features	Analysis
There were no scars on the abdomen, which was not distended. There was no tenderness or guarding. The liver and spleen were not enlarged and there was no mass or evidence of ascites. The groins and genitalia were normal. Rectal examination was normal and there was no blood or melaena.	It is common to have no abnormalities on abdominal examination. Blood has not had time to reach the rectum, suggesting a long transit time or short duration of bleeding.
The casualty officer who had done his preliminary assessment had inserted a large bore intravenous cannula, taken blood for tests and infused plasma protein fraction. The patient continued to be monitored closely.	As mentioned above, resuscitation must be commenced early and full assessment completed later.

Clinical diagnosis

The most likely diagnosis in this patient is peptic ulcer. In favour of this diagnosis are his age, sex, the history of epigastric pain, sometimes nocturnal and eased by antacids, smoking and the absence of features to suggest other diseases.

Endoscopic diagnosis

Bleeding duodenal ulcer was confirmed on endoscopy the following day. There was a large amount of blood and clots in the stomach. The patient was treated by blood transfusion and ulcer healing medications, and his bleeding did not recur. He was advised to give up smoking and to reduce his consumption of alcohol.

Reference

Bailey, H. (1988) *Emergency Surgery*. 11th Edition. John Wright & Sons, Bristol.

Chapter 6

Lower gastrointestinal symptoms

These are grouped together because when a patient presents with any one of them, enquiry should be made about the others. The initial investigations are similar regardless of the symptom the patient complains of. The common symptoms of lower gastrointestinal disease are:

(a) Altered bowel habit
(b) Rectal bleeding
(c) Anal pain
(d) Lump at the anal margin
(e) Prolapse
(f) Itching
(g) Discharge from the anus (other than blood)

Surgical diseases presenting with ano-rectal symptoms (common ones marked *)

Local diseases	*Main presenting symptoms*
Haemorrhoids*	Bleeding, lump at anal verge, pain, itching, discharge
Anal fissure*	Pain, altered bowel habit, bleeding, itching
Anal fistula*	Pain, discharge, lump, itching, bleeding
Perianal abscess*	Pain, lump, discharge
Perianal haematoma	Pain, lump
Diverticular disease	Altered bowel habit, abdominal pain, bleeding
Colorectal cancer*	Altered bowel habit, bleeding, mucus discharge, anaemia
Benign tumours in colon, rectum, anus, e.g. polyps*	Bleeding, discharge, lump at anal verge (for low tumours)
Ulcerative colitis, Crohn's disease*	Bleeding, altered bowel habit
	Note also that anal fissures, fistulae, and abscesses may be a presenting feature of Crohn's disease and ulcerative colitis

97

Local diseases	Main presenting symptoms
Enteric infection	Diarrhoea, bleeding, abdominal pain
Pilonidal sinus*	Pain, discharge, lump in natal cleft (patient often hairy)
Oral antibiotic treatment	Diarrhoea, pruritus
Laxative abuse*	Diarrhoea, discharge (if diarrhoea profuse, patient may have weakness from low potassium)
Rectal prolapse	Prolapse, discharge, itching, altered bowel habit
Infection following anal intercourse (e.g. gonorrhoea, AIDS)	Discharge, bleeding, itching, ulceration, diarrhoea
Anal warts	Pruritus, bleeding

Note that pruritus can occur in diseases such as uraemia, diabetes and jaundice.

Commonest diseases presenting with ano-rectal symptoms.	Haemorrhoids (60%), anal fissure (10%), perianal abscess (7%), anal fistula (5%), ulcerative colitis (5%), Crohn's disease (3%), anal condylomata (3%), laxative abuse (3%), colorectal cancer (3%).
Others	Enteric infections are common but are generally self limiting and rarely present to the surgeon. Nonetheless, the student should be aware of them. Always enquire about travel abroad.

A word about haemorrhoids

Haemorrhoids (or piles) are common and can coexist with other lesions such as malignancy. If a patient presents with rectal bleeding and is found to have haemorrhoids, be sure the bleeding is due to the haemorrhoids. The following are in favour of haemorrhoids: blood bright red in colour; blood on toilet paper and on the outside of the stool rather than mixed with it; no alteration of bowel habit and no loss of appetite or weight; young age: rectal bleeding more likely to be due to haemorrhoids in 20–40 age group than malignancy. Malignancy can occur in this age group. It is always important to exclude higher lesions.

History

Reason for question	Question asked	Comment
Altered bowel habit *Establish normal bowel habit.*	When were your bowels last regular? Describe to me your *normal* bowel habit: Let us take a typical week, on which days would your bowels open? What are your motions normally like? Are they solid/soft/hard? What colour are your motions? When you normally pass your motions, do you have to strain? How long would it take you to evacuate your bowel? Do you take anything for your bowels?	This helps you appreciate the degree of alteration of the bowels

Reason for question	Question asked	Comment
	If so, what, how much and how often? Are you taking more of your usual laxative to keep your bowels working?	Laxative abuse is much more common than is often imagined, and is a frequent cause of diarrhoea
Find out more about altered bowel habit and how it is affecting patient	How did the alteration of your bowels start? Was it related to a specific event such as an unusual food or going abroad? Describe your bowel habit since it became altered: again, take a typical week, describe what happens each day What are your motions like now: liquid, semi-solid, solid, hard?	If the patient uses words like 'diarrhoea', 'constipation', or 'stubborn bowels' ask him to tell you exactly what he means. It is best to describe his bowel pattern, stool frequency, consistency, etc.
	Describe what you see in your stools: blood, slime, undigested food	
	Do the motions flush easily or do they float? Are they particularly smelly?	Think of steatorrhoea
	In what way is your altered bowel habit affecting you? (For instance do you get pain while you pass your motions, does your tummy bloat or hurt, is your back passage itchy etc.?)	

Are these symptoms getting better, worse or are they staying the same?

Intermittent bouts of constipation interrupted by diarrhoea suggest mechanical bowel obstruction due to carcinoma or diverticular disease

Diarrhoea is due to liquefaction of stools above the stenosis

Rectal bleeding
Find out about the quantity, frequency of occurrence etc.

When did you first notice blood in your motions?

Since then, how many times have you seen blood?

How much blood do you see each time: spoonful, egg-cupful, etc?

Is the blood on its own, does it coat the stools, or is it mixed with them?

Or is the blood just on the toilet paper?

Blood on its own or streaking the stool may be due to a low lesion: in anus, e.g. haemorrhoids, or in rectum, e.g. polyps or carcinoma

If the stools are evenly mixed with blood, bleeding is probably coming from higher up, for instance from a sigmoid carcinoma or from diverticular disease

What is the colour of the blood? Is it, for instance, the colour of blood you have when you cut yourself? Or is it darker? How dark?

Bright red blood suggests a low bleeding source such as haemorrhoids or even a carcinoma of the rectum. Dark blood is often from higher up. It is typical of carcinoma

101

Reason for question	Question asked	Comment
	Are your stools black and tarry?	Melaena usually indicates upper GIT bleeding. But note that iron tablets can make the stools black
	Have you noticed anything else in your motions apart from blood, for instance slime or pus?	Suggesting inflammatory bowel disease
Anal pain *When does it occur, what are its characteristics?*	When did the pain first start? Was it during pregnancy or childbirth?	Anal fissure and haemorrhoids common in pregnancy and immediately after
	Where exactly is the pain? Is it outside the anus or inside?	Pain outside the anus may be due to an external lesion such as a perianal abscess
	What brings the pain on? Is it defecation? If so, explain to me exactly what happens when you pass your motions	A painful lesion in the anal canal such as a fissure produces pain when the stool is passing through the anal canal, and the pain is present for some hours afterwards
	Describe the pain. How severe is it?	Pain of fissure is described as throbbing and it is severe

Lump at the anal margin and prolapse

Distinguish between lumps persistently present at the anal margin and those which appear intermittently.

When did you first notice the lump?

How big was it? Show me with one finger exactly where the lump is

What has happened to it since you first noticed it? Has it got bigger, smaller or has it stayed the same?

What makes the lump appear? Opening your bowels?

When it appears after you have your bowels open, does it stay out, or does it pop back up? Does it go back of its own accord or do you have to push it back? Does it come out even if you are not having a bowel motion?

Is it a pilonidal sinus or abscess, for instance?

Think of haemorrhoids or polyps. The grading of haemorrhoids depends on this property. Those which never prolapse are referred to as first degree; those which appear when the patient strains or defecates, but return spontaneously after or can be reduced manually, are second degree. Those which are permanently prolapsed and cannot be reduced at all are third degree

Itching

Is it local itching or does the patient itch elsewhere?

When did the itching start?

Have you any idea what might have started it? for instance some tablets, a food, a cream?

Where do you itch? Just around the back passage or elsewhere?

If elsewhere, show me where. In women, any itching around the front passage or the vagina?

Suggesting an allergic cause

Think of local causes such as anal warts; or disease in neighbouring organs such as in the genital tract; or elsewhere in the bowel, for instance due to excessive use of liquid paraffin; or to generalized disorder, for example jaundice or diabetes

103

Reason for question	Question asked	Comment
Discharge from the anus (other than blood)		
Establish nature of discharge.	Questions almost exactly as for bleeding per rectum.	Purulent discharge in proctitis, e.g. ulcerative or gonococcal. Mucus in colitis, carcinoma and haemorrhoids
REVIEW OF SYSTEMS	*Finish rest of GIT*	Remember possibility of disease elsewhere in the GIT producing ano-rectal symptoms
	RS, GUS, CNS, CVS	If malignancy is suspected think of spread to other organs such as lung or brain
PMH	Diabetes, previous perianal disease, Crohn's disease, ulcerative colitis	
FH		
SH	Enquire about patient's sexual orientation	It is important to think of receptive anal intercourse as a cause of perianal symptoms
DRUGS	*Enquire about laxative use* Anti-Parkinsonian agents	These are among a number of drugs that cause constipation
ALLERGIES		Pruritus may be due to allergy

Examination

Reason for examination	*Sign elicited*	*Comment*
General examination	Age: think of colorectal cancer in a patient over the age of 50 presenting with change in bowel habit and/or rectal bleeding but remember that it can occur even in younger patients. If you suspect malignancy, look for signs of it on general examination: cachexia, anaemia, jaundice, enlarged lymph nodes in the neck.	
	Any skin lesions such as eczema	Suggesting allergic cause for pruritus
RS	Any signs of lung collapse, consolidation or effusion?	Signs of secondary carcinoma in the lungs
CVS, CNS		
ABDOMEN	Distension with shifting dullness	This may be malignant ascites in a patient with cancer
	Mass	Consider primary carcinoma in the colon
	Enlarged liver	Possibility of secondary deposits in the liver
Signs of intestinal obstruction	Resonance of abdomen to percussion, distension, hyperactive and continuous bowel sounds	These are features of intestinal obstruction. Think of a colonic neoplasm
	Inguinal lymph nodes	The possibilities are spread from anal carcinoma, perianal infection

Reason for examination	Sign elicited	Comment
RECTAL EXAMINATION	This is the most important part of the examination. Many diseases will be diagnosed simply by careful inspection. Make sure the patient is comfortable in the left lateral position and that the light is good. If you find an unusual lesion at the anal margin, think of Crohn's disease or ulcerative colitis as a cause.	
	Inspection: Natal cleft	Any evidence of pilonidal sinus?
	Faecal soiling, state of cleanliness of perianal area	Ano-rectal symptoms may be due to poor hygiene or to incontinence
	Any rash or other skin lesion?	
	Scar: from previous ano-rectal operation such as drainage of abscess	
	Think of each of the following lesions and look for evidence of:	
	Anal warts:	
	Abscess: swelling and redness	
	Perianal sinus: external opening of sinus	
	Fistula-in-ano: external opening of fistula	
	Fissure: tight anal sphincter; sentinel anal tag	Fissure is the commonest cause of anal spasm
	The fissure can sometimes be seen if the buttocks are parted gently	
	Haemorrhoids: prolapsed piles	
	Carcinoma: anal carcinoma, lower edge of rectal carcinoma or rectal polyp	
	Rectal prolapse: ask the patient to strain to see if the prolapse occurs	

Palpation: As for inspection this must be systematic, and specific diseases should be borne in mind:

The perianal area: tenderness over abscess or near fissure; induration over fistula tract and discharge from its external opening

Anal canal: induration of anal fistula tract. Note that haemorrhoids are not normally palpable. Can the finger be introduced easily, or is the sphincter tight?

The sphincter is tight following a haemorrhoid operation in which excessive perianal tissue is removed. Pain and spasm of anal sphincter also make digital (and instrumental) rectal examination excruciating for the patient

Rectum: Any masses must be carefully assessed for position, extent, and whether fixed or mobile

Think of carcinoma of rectum, masses outside the rectum such as tumour deposits in the pouch of Douglas

LOOK AT THE EXAMINING FINGER AFTER IT IS WITHDRAWN: any blood, pus or mucus? What is the character of the stool?

A high tumour may not be palpable but its presence may be suggested by blood. Blood and pus may be due to colitis

Proctoscopy and sigmoidoscopy: These are still part of clinical examination. They are mandatory in all patients presenting with symptoms of lower gastrointestinal disease. Important lesions may be missed if they are not carried out. Proctoscopy allows the anal canal to be examined for haemorrhoids and the internal opening of a fistula. It is often too painful in fissure and must not be performed without anaesthesia. Sigmoidoscopy will show the rectal mucosa and will enable a clinical diagnosis of carcinoma, polyps and inflammatory bowel disease. Suspicious areas are biopsied for histological examination.

Further investigation: If a lesion is found to account for the patient's symptoms, and there is no suspicion of a sinister condition such as malignancy, in many cases further investigation is not needed. If there is any doubt about the diagnosis or if the symptoms continue despite adequate treatment, further investigation should be performed. This is particularly the case with bleeding from haemorrhoids.

Barium enema and colonoscopy: Which one of these investigations is carried out first depends on the facilities available in your hospital, on the expertise of the investigators and on the diagnosis suspected. Barium enema is more widely available than colonoscopy and is therefore requested more often. Colonoscopy is more invasive and requires sedation but has the advantage that it allows direct visualization of the whole colon in expert hands and can reveal small lesions such as polyps easily missed on barium examination. Also, lesions can be biopsied and some, such as polyps, can be excised through the colonoscope.

Case report

Features	Analysis
Mrs Jane Cooper is aged 68. She is widowed and lives alone in her flat 10 minutes'walk from her married daughter's house. She presented to her GP with a 7-month history of 'stubborn bowels' and intermittent rectal bleeding.	Note the patient's age. We must define exactly what she means by 'stubborn bowels'. Similarly, complaints such as 'diarrhoea' and 'constipation' must not be accepted without clear description. Rectal bleeding requires full investigation. At this age, we must think of malignancy.

She rarely visits her GP, except for occasional check-ups and regular repeat prescriptions for hypertension. She was well and symptom free until 7 months before she noticed these symptoms. Normally, she opened her bowels once every 1 or 2 days and her stools were soft and 'came away easily'. Seven months ago she found that every 2 weeks, she would not open her bowels for three or four days and when she did go, she had to strain to pass stools. This is what she meant by 'stubborn bowels'; for her this was unusual. Over the next 4 months, her bowel frequency gradually changed to one stool every 3 or 4 days.

The 'history of the presenting complaints' gives us the chance to interrogate the patient about her symptoms. Clearly, there has been a change in this lady's bowel habit in that she was going less often than usual and had to strain. Think of a progressively obstructing lesion in the large bowel such as malignancy and diverticular disease.

She first saw blood in her stools 6 months before she presented. It appeared once a month after that. The blood was dark red and was mixed with her stools, and the quantity was approximately 1 teaspoonful per motion. She never passed blood other than with stools, and had not been aware of mucus or pus in the stools.

Dark blood mixed with stools suggests a high lesion such as carcinoma of the sigmoid colon. By contrast, bright red blood on the outside of the stool or seen on toilet paper is typical of a lesion in the anus or lower rectum, most commonly, haemorrhoids.

Her appetite was good and her weight had not changed. She denied abdominal pain, distension and jaundice. She had not noticed any lumps, itching, pain or discharge at the anal verge or in the anus.

Poor appetite and weight loss are ominous symptoms in someone of this age presenting with the above symptoms, for they may be due to secondary tumour. Their absence does not rule out secondaries. Enquire about other GI symptoms.

Features	Analysis
She had no other symptoms on systems review. She was found to be hypertensive 30 years ago and had taken a number of medications over the years. Currently, she was on nifedipine 20 mg twice daily, on which her blood pressure was well controlled. She had had no other illnesses or operations.	It is important to search for intercurrent disease. Her blood pressure appears to be well controlled but she should have an adequate cardiovascular appraisal, especially if an operation is necessary.
She coped well at home with all her daily chores and played bingo at weekends. She did not smoke or drink alcohol. Her father died fighting in the Second World War and her mother died from ischaemic heart disease at the age of 80. There was no history of bowel cancer in the family.	If large bowel cancer is suspected, as in this patient, a detailed family history should be taken. In some individuals, colorectal cancer is familial.
General examination was unremarkable. She was not anaemic or jaundiced, and there were no enlarged nodes in the neck. Examination of the heart and lungs revealed no abnormalities. BP was 140/85, pulse 72/min and regular and all peripheral pulses were normal.	These normal findings are encouraging in the search for other diseases and for secondaries if cancer found.
There were no scars on the abdomen, which was not distended. There was no tenderness and no masses. The liver and spleen were not palpable, and bowel sounds were normal. There were no palpable groin nodes or hernias.	Clinical examination of the abdomen is normal. This of course does not rule out intra-abdominal disease.

Rectal examination showed soft brown stools and no blood, and there were no masses or tenderness. Proctoscopy showed small internal haemorrhoids.

Lower limbs were normal.

The haemorrhoids are unlikely to be the cause of the rectal bleeding. As explained above, the blood is more likely to have come from a higher lesion.

Clinical diagnosis
The two lesions that commonly cause a change in bowel habit and rectal bleeding in a woman of this age with no previous GI symptoms are carcinoma of the large bowel and diverticular disease. Diverticular disease is common at this age but malignancy must be excluded.

Sigmoidoscopy
This was performed in the clinic and showed an ulcerated mass in the lower sigmoid colon. Biopsies were taken and histology showed a moderately differentiated invasive adenocarcinoma.

Further investigations
Colonoscopy confirmed the sigmoidoscopic findings, and it showed, in addition, diverticular disease in the sigmoid colon. There were no other lesions in the large bowel. Chest X-ray and ultrasound of the abdomen were normal, as were blood count and LFTs.

Final diagnosis
Carcinoma of the lower sigmoid colon with involved mesenteric lymph nodes. There were no liver secondaries.

Chapter 7

Anorexia, lethargy and weight loss

Sometimes the surgeon is asked to investigate patients with chronic symptoms which cannot be immediately attributed to disease in a particular organ or system. If a major localizing symptom such as dysphagia is present, the investigation should be directed to it. Such non-specific symptoms, common in general practice, may be due to physical or psychiatric illness, or combinations of these, but in many patients, no disease can be found. It must be remembered that these may be the presenting features of some serious disorders, hence full history, examination and investigation are important.

Causes

Physiological derangement	*Physical causes*	
Overwork and inadequate rest	Drugs: diuretics, beta-blockers, alcohol	Metabolic: Diabetes mellitus
Insomnia	Infections: Infectious mononucleosis	Hyperparathyroidism
Lack of physical or mental stimulation	Tuberculosis	Hypothyroidism
	Viral hepatitis	Hyperthyroidism (apathetic type)
Recent illness or operation		
Starvation	Infective endocarditis	Uraemia
Chronic anaemia (from any cause)	Acquired immune deficiency syndrome AIDS	Insulinoma
	Intestinal infestation	

Psychological causes

Anxiety and depression
Psychotic illness   *Malignant neoplasms*, especially those affecting: *Inflammatory disorders:*
Anorexia nervosa   Stomach   Connective tissue disorders
Bulimia   Pancreas
                                                Bronchus
                                                Lymphoreticular system

Commoner causes   For the surgeon the most important groups of causes are those due to malignant and
                                            metabolic diseases, but overall the physiological derangements and psychological
                                            causes are the most common. In many patients, no definite cause will be found.

Points to look for

The clinical history will show evidence of physiological disturbances such as fatigue, inadequate rest, or of recent illness or operation. It may disclose localizing symptoms which the patient may have disregarded, or it may identify factors that suggest a specific cause. For instance, if a middle-aged patient has in addition to the presenting symptoms a history of recent epigastric pain, carcinoma of the pancreas or stomach should be considered in the diagnosis. Iatrogenic causes such as treatment with beta-blockers and diuretics and abuse of drugs and alcohol must be excluded. Psychiatric disease must be diagnosed on positive evidence rather than merely by excluding physical illness.

Surgical diagnoses that must be considered include the following:

Carcinoma of the stomach

The onset of anorexia, malaise and weight loss,

113

especially if associated with epigastric pain of recent onset in a middle-aged or elderly patient, must alert you to the possibility of carcinoma of the stomach. There may be profound depression and the patient may be pale, ill and malnourished. There may be no other physical signs but in later stages there may be enlarged lymph nodes in the neck and an abdominal mass or ascites. Unfortunately, carcinoma of the stomach frequently presents late especially if the lesion is in the fundus or the body of the stomach. Lesions in the pylorus are more likely to produce pyloric stenosis.

Carcinoma of the body of the pancreas

Neoplasms in the head of the pancreas obstruct the common bile duct and produce obstructive jaundice in 65% of patients afflicted. Tumours in the body or the tail of the pancreas often present, or are diagnosed, only when the disease is advanced. The patient complains of abdominal pain and backache in addition to the non-specific symptoms under discussion. Sometimes, the patient presents with metastases (especially hepatic) and no symptoms from the primary tumour.

History

Reason for question	Question asked	Comment
Establish previous health and duration of symptoms.	When were you last well and free of these symptoms? For how long have you felt unwell and tired?	Symptoms of recent onset may be due to physiological or physical causes. Malignant disease must be considered if the patient has lost much weight. Suspect psychiatric illness if symptoms have been present for more than a year

*Discover predominant
symptom and its
progression.*

Which of the your complaints is troubling you
most?
How has it progressed over the last few weeks,
months or years?

Any of the symptoms, if progressing and
deteriorating rapidly with time, should raise
the possibility of physical illness, especially
malignant disease or diabetes

Weight loss and anorexia
(See Introduction for questions to ask to
determine amount of weight lost)

*Determine whether
weight loss is
physiological or due
to physical causes.
Work out food intake*

Why do you think you are losing weight?
What is your appetite like?
How much are you eating? Take a typical week;
tell me the meals you eat each day and what
they contain. Do you eat any other foods?
Do you drink alcohol, if so how many units
a week?

It is important to get the patient's opinion on
the reason for his weight loss. It may be due
for example, to excessive dieting
Reduced food intake is often the result of
anorexia but may be due to poverty or
dislike for food, or inability to chew or
swallow, or to vomiting

*Question about energy
usage*

Please tell me about your daily activities
How much physical exercise do you do, at
home, at work and during your leisure?

Weight loss in spite of adequate food intake
should raise suspicion about diabetes,
hyperthyroidism or insulinoma
Although weight loss may indicate malignant
disease, steady weight or even weight gain
may be observed in some patients with
cancer. The amount of weight lost does not
correlate with the stage of the tumour

Reason for question	Question asked	Comment
Enquire about energy loss	*How are your bowels?* *Do you vomit?*	Diarrhoea and vomiting may be reason for weight loss
	Lethargy How much energy do you have for work, housework and for your hobbies?	The localizing value of this symptom is poor. It may be due to weight loss, starvation or muscle wasting, and it may accompany all the causes listed above
Find out about associated symptoms Nausea/vomiting	Have you felt sick or been sick? (nausea or vomiting).	Vomiting may be due to mechanical bowel obstruction, for instance from carcinoma of the stomach
Fever/rigors	Have you felt hot and shivery? (fever and rigors)	Fever and rigors suggest an infective cause, especially TB in those most at risk. Hodgkin's disease must also be considered
Sleep	Do you sleep well?	Insomnia may be a cause of the symptoms; alternatively, it may be a consequence of illness, especially depression
Weather preference	Do you have a preference for any particular weather?	Consider hyperthyroidism or hypothyroidism as a cause of symptoms. If so, enquire in more detail about thyroid status as in Chapter 9

ROS

Systems review is important as it may enable localization of the symptoms to an organ or system. GIT	GIT: Dysphagia	Possibility of carcinoma of the oesophagus
	Epigastric pain	Carcinoma of the stomach or of the pancreas must be thought of in a middle-aged or elderly patient who presents with a short history of epigastric pain (less than 6 months)
	Jaundice	This suggests secondary carcinoma of the liver or carcinoma in the biliary tree or in the pancreas
	Diarrhoea	May be due to carcinoma of the large bowel or inflammatory bowel disease, especially if blood is present in the stools. Infestation of the bowel must also be considered, especially if the patient has recently come from abroad
	Constipation	Think of mechanical bowel obstruction, for instance due to carcinoma; of hyperparathyroidism; or drugs
CVS	Angina and dyspnoea	These may be secondary to anaemia or cardiac disease
RS	Cough, sputum, haemoptysis	Consider bronchogenic carcinoma

117

Reason for question	Question asked	Comment
GUS	Loin pain, ureteric colic, fever and rigors, disturbances of micturition, haematuria	Carcinoma or TB of the urinary tract should be thought of
CNS	Forgetfulness, confusion, coma, fits	Metabolic disturbances such as uraemia, and diabetes. In a patient who has arrived from abroad, think of malaria
Psychiatric history	Change in social or personal circumstances which may have caused depression, e.g. bereavement, redundancy	A diagnosis of psychiatric disorder must be based on positive evidence and not merely on the exclusion of physical disease
	Premorbid personality, mood, intellect, will; delusions	
PMH Cardiac disease	Heart failure, ischaemic heart disease	Heart failure and treatment with diuretics and beta-blockers can produce chronic symptoms listed above
Operations	Recent operation or acute illness, especially infection	Physiological reaction or the effect of recent infective illness
Thyroidectomy	Previous thyroidectomy	The risk of hypothyroidism depends on the reason for thyroidectomy and the amount of thyroid left behind. It is high following subtotal thyroidectomy for thyrotoxicosis

Malignant disease	Previous treatment for malignant disease	Consider possibility of recurrence
Diabetes	Diabetes mellitus	The disease may be poorly controlled
FH	Mental illness, malignant disease, ischaemic heart disease	
SH	Recent travel abroad or emigration. Note alcohol intake and habit	Infectious disease, alcohol and smoking and smoking-related illnesses may cause the symptoms
	Occupation: satisfaction with work; redundancy; overwork; inadequate rest; lack of motivation	
	Change in social circumstances	
	Drug abuse	
DRUGS	Especially beta-blockers and diuretics	
ALLERGIES		

Examination

Reason for examination	Sign elicited	Comment
General	Patients with depressive illness are often well but may look apathetic and sad. If the patient is unwell and undernourished, consider the possibility of infection or malignant disease. Patients with physiological disturbance, for instance, those deprived of sleep, look exhausted but are well. Remember that patients with chronic renal failure may present with anorexia, weight loss and lethargy, and few other features.	
	Pallor (look also for glossitis and koilonychia)	Anaemia sometimes occurs with chronic infections, inflammatory disorders, neoplasms and malnutrition. Anaemia from any cause may itself be responsible for these symptoms
	Check temperature	There may be fever in inflammatory and infective illnesses, and in Hodgkin's disease but it is often intermittent
	Jaundice	May be present with carcinoma, infections and inflammations
	Enlarged lymph nodes	Think of TB, malignancy including lymphoma, connective tissue disorders, AIDS
	Note skin texture, rash or joint stiffness	Consider connective tissue disorders
RS	Look for signs of lung collapse, consolidation, pleural effusion	Respiratory signs (see introduction) may be due to TB, pneumonia, primary lung cancer or secondaries

CVS	Look for evidence of heart disease, e.g. arrhythmias, raised JVP, crackles, heart murmurs, displaced apex beat, gallop rhythm, etc.	Heart failure is an important cause of lethargy. Hypertension may be due to chronic renal failure
CNS	Impairment of consciousness and other neurological abnormalities	Impairment of consciousness may be due to metabolic derangements and chronic infections
ABDOMEN	Scars	Previous operations for cancer
	Distension	May be due to ascites or intestinal obstruction from malignant disease
	Masses	These may be due to intra-abdominal malignancy
	Enlarged liver	Think of secondary carcinoma, hepatitis and cirrhosis
	Ano-rectal examination looking for fissures, fistulae, masses, blood in rectum	If present, these raise the possibility of inflammatory bowel disease or carcinoma of rectum
PSYCHIATRIC EXAMINATION	Level of consciousness, intellect, mood, will/drive, reality testing, personality	There may be evidence of psychiatric illness to account for symptoms

Investigations

Urinalysis: This may show glycosuria due to diabetes mellitus. The presence of bilirubin and urobilinogen should suggest biliary obstruction from liver disease (e.g. hepatitis), biliary tract and pancreatic disorders (e.g. carcinoma of the pancreas). In children and elderly patients, MSU should be sent for culture, as this may reveal urinary tract infection. In immigrant patients, tuberculosis must be considered and if the chest X-ray is normal, it may be necessary to send urine for culture for TB.

Hb, WCC, ESR or CRP: These should be requested and may show anaemia. Anaemia may be responsible for the symptoms, or it may itself be due to an underlying disorder such as leukaemia, carcinoma or connective tissue disorder. ESR is non-specific but if it is abnormally high, further investigations will be necessary to find the cause.

Blood urea and electrolytes: Uraemia may be the cause of the patient's symptoms.

LFTs: These may be abnormal in liver, biliary and pancreatic disorders. Raised calcium may be due to hyperparathyroidism or to secondary carcinoma in bone.

Thyroid function tests: Remember that classic features of hyperthyroidism are not always present.

Chest X-ray: Carcinoma of the bronchus is a common malignancy and must be sought or excluded. If chest symptoms and signs present, a chest X-ray should be performed.

Other investigations depend on the history and the examination. If, for example, carcinoma of the stomach is suspected, barium meal or gastroscopy should be performed. If the liver is found to be enlarged or if the liver function tests are abnormal, ultrasound scan of the upper abdomen must be performed.

Case report

Features	*Analysis*
Mr Pramod Johal, a 55-year-old Indian man, is a waiter in a restaurant. He works from 5 p.m. to midnight on week days and until 2 a.m. at weekends. He is happily married and has two grown up children who are accountants. He was referred to the surgical clinic by his general practitioner because of a 5-month history of 'feeling under the weather', weight loss of 8 kg and mild epigastric pain.	Important points to bear in mind in this man's presentation are his age, his ethnic background and of course his symptoms. His astute GP had also referred him to a surgical, and not a medical clinic. Initial diagnoses that spring to mind are carcinoma of the stomach, alcohol abuse, overwork, depression and tuberculosis. However, as always, do not draw conclusions until you have heard the whole story.
Mr Johal had enjoyed good health and was free of symptoms until 5 months ago when he began to feel unwell and lethargic. Business at the restaurant had become particularly brisk over the last 6 months and often he helped on his days off to earn extra money. Before his illness, he would sleep 6 hours after work and then spend the rest of his free time doing DIY jobs in the house or repairing his car, both of which he enjoyed. In the last 5 months he has tended to stay in bed for up to 12 hours and has not had any energy to do his house jobs and car repairs. He wakes up feeling tired and even his work, which he used to enjoy doing, was becoming difficult. He weighed himself regularly and noticed he had lost 8 kg in 5 months, but he had not been dieting. His appetite had diminished but he managed to eat well.	The onset of these symptoms in a previously well man deserves full investigation. This amount of weight loss should arouse concern. Attention should rightly focus on his occupation and there is a firm possibility that his symptoms are due to overwork. A full psychiatric history is also mandatory in a man who loses interest in his job and hobbies, and presents with weight loss.

Features	*Analysis*
He complained of intermittent upper abdominal pain not related to food. He denied dysphagia, vomiting, jaundice or alteration of his bowel habits. He had woken up from sleep on several occasions with fever and rigors. There were no other symptoms on systems review. In particular he had no cough, sputum or haemoptysis. He had smoked 5 cigarettes a day for 10 years but did not drink alcohol or use illicit drugs. There were no features to suggest depression.	Systems review is important in a case such as this, for it begins to give us our first clues that this man's symptoms are due to organic disease. Epigastric pain suggests carcinoma of the stomach or benign peptic ulcer. Fever and rigors should alert you to think of Hodgkin's disease and tuberculosis, the latter in view view of his race. Also think of malaria if there are no other symptoms.
He was well but looked tired and pale. He was not jaundiced. There was a single, large and firm node in his left supraclavicular fossa. The thyroid was not palpable and the chest was clear. Abdominal, rectal examination, locomotor and neurological examination were normal.	This lymph node is clearly pathological. The diagnoses to consider now are carcinoma of the stomach, Hodgkin's disease and tuberculosis.

Clinical diagnosis
Weight loss, lethargy, epigastric pain and the left supraclavicular node in a man of 55 should make you think of carcinoma of the stomach (see Chapters 1 and 2). In favour of Hodgkin's disease and TB are weight loss, lethargy, fever and sweating, and the enlarged lymph node.

Investigations

Examination of the ears, nose and throat by an ENT specialist did not show any disease in these areas.	This examination is mandatory before biopsy of neck lymph nodes in adults (see Chapter 8–investigations).

124

Lymph node biopsy showed features of TB and acid and alcohol fast bacilli were seen.

This confirms the diagnosis of TB. The patient was commenced on anti-tuberculous therapy.

A portion of lymph node was sent for culture and the results were available later.
Mycobacterium tuberculosis was cultured and its antibiotic sensitivities determined.

The combination drugs can be altered if proved by culture to be wrong.

Chest X-ray was normal.

It is common to find patients with glandular TB who have weight loss but no evidence of pulmonary TB.

Barium meal and upper gastrointestinal endoscopy in this patient were normal.

It was important in this patient to rule out carcinoma of the stomach. It is likely that this patient's abdominal pain was due to intra-abdominal TB; it cleared with anti-tuberculous treatment.

Hb was 9.4 g/dl with a normochromic and normocytic blood picture. ESR was grossly elevated at 120 mm in the first hour.

This blood picture is in keeping with the diagnosis. It should be monitored and should improve with successful treatment of the disease.

Chapter 8

Lumps in the neck (other than in thyroid)

Anatomical considerations

The midline of the neck is defined by an imaginary line drawn from the symphysis menti (the point of fusion of the two halves of the mandible) through the notch of the thyroid cartilage to the middle of the suprasternal notch (Fig 8.1). On either side, the neck is divided into anterior and posterior triangles by the sternomastoid muscle. The base of the anterior triangle points upwards, while that of the posterior triangle points downwards. The anterior triangle has at its upper end a subsidiary triangle known as the digastric triangle the lower border of which is formed by the digastric muscle. At the lower end of the posterior triangle is a smaller triangle known as the supraclavicular fossa, the upper margin of which is the posterior belly of the omohyoid muscle. The investing layer of deep cervical fascia splits to enclose the sternomastoid and divides each triangle into a superficial and deep plane. The relation of a mass to the deep fascia can be determined by contracting the sternomastoid muscle: this is done by getting the

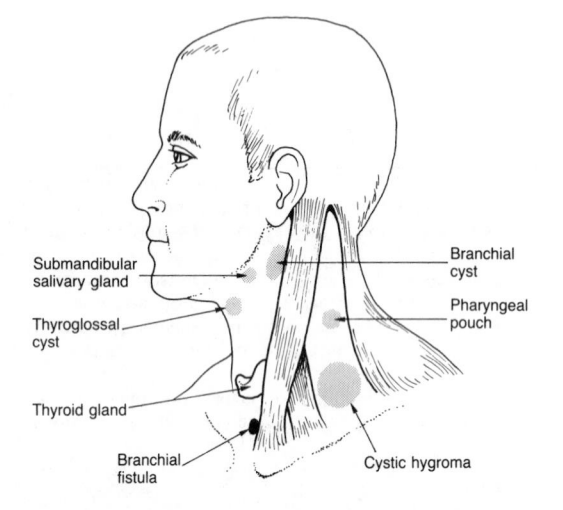

Figure 8.1. *The triangles of the neck and the common surgical disorders that affect them. Lymph nodes are omitted*

patient to push his chin down against the resistance of your hand. If the lump is in the superficial plane it will still be palpable, whereas a lump in the deep plane will be felt less easily.

Lumps and ulcers arising in the plane superficial to the deep cervical fascia can occur elsewhere in the body. These include sebaceous cysts, lipomata and basal cell carcinomas. Lymph nodes can occur in either plane.

Classification of lumps in the neck

Masses in the neck can arise either from unpaired midline structures (the masses may not be exactly in the midline, but may lie a little to one or other side), or from paired lateral structures (Fig 8.1).

Masses from unpaired midline structures	*Masses arising from paired lateral structures*
1. Thyroglossal cyst 2. Lumps from the isthmus of the thyroid gland	1. Lymph nodes 2. Branchial cyst 3. Lumps from the thyroid gland 4. Submandibular salivary gland swellings (in digastric triangle) 5. Pharyngeal pouch (lies in posterior triangle) 6. Cervical rib 7. Aneurysms of the neck arteries 8. Cystic hygroma

Commonest causes of swelling in neck other than thyroid

The commonest are lymph nodes (80%) and salivary gland swellings (7%). Pharyngeal pouch and thyroglossal cyst account for less than 2%.

Points to look for

Lymph node enlargement is due most often to transient infection of the upper respiratory tract, the mouth and the pharynx and larynx. Secondary spread of tumour from elsewhere to the neck is the next commonest cause of lymphadenopathy. Other causes which must be considered are malignancies of the lymphoid and blood forming cells (e.g. lymphoma and leukaemia) and chronic infections, especially tuberculosis and infectious mononucleosis (glandular fever). Think of tuberculosis in immigrants, especially from the Third World.

Lump arising from unpaired midline structures

Thyroglossal cyst

The thyroid gland develops from a duct, the foramen caecum, at the junction of the anterior two-thirds and posterior third of the tongue. The duct passes downwards in the midline from this foramen and lies close to the hyoid bone. From here, it passes to the position of the isthmus where the two lobes grow outwards. Failure of any part of this duct to obliterate causes a thyroglossal cyst. These cysts are found most commonly at the lower border of the hyoid bone, and lie slightly to one side of the midline. Smaller cysts may not fluctuate, and many transilluminate. Because of

their relation to the hyoid bone, these cysts will move when the tongue is protruded. Hold the patient's mouth open and ask him to protrude his tongue. The cyst will move or tug upwards.

Lump arising from paired lateral structures

Lymph nodes

These are the commonest swellings in the neck and are dealt with in the text.

Branchial cyst

The remnant of the branchial cleft (usually the second), when present, runs from the oropharynx to the skin of the anterior triangle of the neck. It opens just in front of the anterior border of the sterno-mastoid muscle half way down the neck. The whole of the cleft may be patent and results in a branchial fistula. More often, however, the deeper end is obliterated to form a branchial sinus which discharges clear fluid on to the skin, or the two ends may be closed off to form a branchial cyst.

A branchial cyst occurs in a young patient who is usually less than 40 years of age. Its deep margin cannot be identified, and the swelling is soft and fluctuant. It does not usually transilluminate because of its deep position. If inflamed it may be tender to touch.

Submandibular salivary gland

As for other salivary glands, the submandibular gland may become enlarged because of non-specific inflammation, mumps, obstruction of the duct, and tumours. The symptoms which accompany the swelling will depend on the disease: pain with infection or duct obstruction. The pain of duct obstruction characteristically comes on during meals when the flow of saliva is stimulated. In this case the gland will be tender on palpation. Neoplasms present as a painless lump which may vary in consistency from soft to firm and hard. The gland is roughly oval in shape but its surface is irregular. It is best palpated bimanually with the index finger of one hand in the mouth and two fingers of the other hand outside beneath the jaw. The duct should also be palpated for calculi from the gland to the orifice on one side of the tongue. The duct orifice should be inspected by asking the patient to lift his tongue: if a stone is impacted it will be visible through the stretched orifice.

Pharyngeal pouch

There is a triangular gap at the back of the inferior constrictor of the pharynx between the upper border of the transversely running fibres of the cricopharyngeal muscle below and the lower border of the obliquely running fibres of the thyropharyngeal above. Through this gap, known as the dehiscence of Killian, the mucosa of the pharynx bulges to form a pharyngeal pouch. This pouch gradually expands and bulges into the neck, usually on the left hand side, and lies in the posterior triangle behind the sternomastoid muscle. The first symptom is regurgitation of undigested food, which the patient may recognize he had eaten many days before. At this stage the lump is vague, but as it enlarges, it can be felt. It presses on the oesophagus and causes dysphagia. He may also notice some gurgling sounds in his neck. Dysphagia leads to weight loss.

The swelling is in the posterior triangle behind the deep fascia, and its margins are indistinct. If compressed it can be emptied. The lungs must be examined for evidence of aspiration pneumonia. This is likely to have taken place if there is collapse, consolidation or bronchopneumonia.

Aneurysm

As with arteries elsewhere, the large arteries in the neck can become aneurysmal, although this is rare. More often they are simply tortuous. The vessels affected are the cervical part of the subclavian or the carotid arteries. In the carotids they may give rise to reduced blood flow to the brain (causing permanent neurological deficits) or to embolism (causing transient ischaemic cerebral attacks). There is dilatation of the vessel and the swelling is pulsatile. Auscultate for bruits.

An approach to swellings in the neck

If you are asked to examine a patient with a swelling or other lesion in the neck, you can save yourself much time by doing a quick preliminary examination before you begin taking the history in detail. Answer three questions:

1. Is the lesion in the thyroid gland or outside it?

Give the patient a glass of water and ask him to take some of the water in his mouth. Ask the patient to lift up his chin and then to swallow the water. If the lump moves upwards when the patient swallows, the lump is in the thyroid. Proceed as for thyroid lumps in Chapter 9; otherwise go to 2 below.

2. Is it a thyroglossal cyst?

For a lesion in the midline or close to it, ask the patient to open his mouth and to protrude his tongue steadily. If the lump is a thyroglossal cyst attached to the hyoid bone, it will rise in the neck or it will tug upwards. Take a history and examine as for any lump, enquiring about duration, pain and increase in size (suggesting infection in the cyst), etc. Thyroglossal cysts lie near the midline, between the symphysis menti and the upper border of the isthmus of the thyroid gland. Many will fluctuate and some will transilluminate. The examination is not complete until you have examined the base of the tongue for a lingual thyroid, for embryologically the thyroid arises at the base of the tongue and migrates into the neck. A lingual thyroid has the appearance of a piece of red tissue applied to the base of the tongue. It is rare.

3. Is it possibly a lymph node?

Nodes are often lateral; discrete; firm, soft or hard; and mobile. Most cervical nodes lie just in front of and deep to the anterior border of the sternomastoid muscle. Others may be in the preauricular or occipital area and in the posterior triangle.

If you discover a lymph node or nodes in the neck, you must try to establish the underlying cause, for instance infection or malignancy in the upper respiratory tract, especially the nasopharynx, or elsewhere (see below). Examine also other node-bearing areas such as the axillae and groins. Do not forget to examine the liver and spleen, which may be enlarged in certain diseases manifesting with peripheral lymph node enlargement (below).

The causes of lymph node enlargement are:

Infection: tonsillitis, TB, infectious mononucleosis, AIDS.

Malignancy: 10% primary, 80% metastatic squamous carcinoma, 10% other metastases. Of metastatic squamous tumours, 90% are from primaries in the head and neck. Remember lymphomas and thyroid cancers, and tumours from the chest and abdomen, and testis in men.

Others: sarcoidosis.

History

Reason for question	Question asked	Comment
Duration of lesion	When did you first notice the lump in your neck? What brought this swelling to your attention? Has it changed in size? By how much, and over how long?	Lumps which have been present for a long time and which are only growing slowly are probably benign
Associated symptoms	What problems has it caused: Pain?	Suggests inflammation or infection, for example, enlarged nodes due to infection or obstructed submandibular gland by calculus
	Gurgling noises in your neck or difficulty with swallowing?	Suggest a pharyngeal pouch
Multiple lesions	Are there any other lumps like this anywhere else?	Lymph nodes are often multiple. The may all be in the cervical region or they may be in other node-bearing areas
If lump is a lymph node, what caused it?	Any sore throat, ear ache, headaches, runny nose, sore eyes?	Symptoms of upper respiratory infection
	Enquire about weight loss, malaise, anorexia, lethargy	Non-specific symptoms of neoplasia or chronic infection
	Any fever and night sweats?	Think of tuberculosis or Hodgkin's disease

132

ROS	CVS, CNS, RS, GUS, GIT	This will give a clue to patient's general health, the existence of systemic disease such as chronic infection or neoplasia
PMH	Enquire about treatment for malignant disease	Swelling may be a lymph node suggesting recurrence or secondary deposit
FH, SH, DRUGS ALLERGIES		

Examination

Reason for examination	*Sign elicited*	*Comment*
General examination	If lymph node(s) found, look for general signs of malignancy. Patients with malignant disease or chronic infection such as TB may look ill and may have lost weight. Anaemia may be due to chronic infection such as TB or to malignant disease, especially leukaemia. There may be pyrexia in acute infection such as tonsillitis.	
Local examination	The diagnostic possibilities are few. Take each one in turn and do specific examination to see if it is present. Preliminary examination should have been done to exclude thyroid swelling or thyroglossal cyst.	
Lymph node(s)	Determine site, size, number, tissue plane in which present, etc. as for any lump (see Introduction).	

Reason for examination	Sign elicited	Comment
Look for site of primary disease	Examine scalp, ears, nose, mouth, throat, salivary glands, thyroid, breasts	Look for evidence of acute or chronic infection or of neoplasia at all of these sites
Clues from location of node	The location of a lymph node will give an indication of the site of the primary infection or malignant neoplasm: Pre-auricular node – scalp, face, ear, parotid gland Submental node – front of floor of mouth, tip of tongue, centre of lower lip, mandible Submandibular node – mouth, facial bone sinuses, cheek, nose, lips High jugular node – facial bone sinuses, nose, pharynx, larynx. In particular, look at tonsils, and base of tongue Mid-jugular node – thyroid, pharynx, larynx, submandibular salivary gland Low jugular node – thyroid, upper oesophagus, thorax, upper abdomen Supraclavicular – chest, abdomen (including testis), breast, upper limb	
Clues from other properties of node	Tenderness and signs of inflammation over node suggest acute infection such as tonsillitis A hard node, especially if fixed, should make you think of secondary carcinoma or TB If the node is rubbery, consider lymphoma, especially Hodgkin's disease	
Branchial cyst	Described above	
Submandibular salivary gland	Any signs of overlying inflammation? This suggests infection of gland or obstruction of duct by stone If firm or fixed think of malignancy	

Pharyngeal pouch	Described above	
Thyroglossal cyst	Excluding the thyroid, the five lesions here account for nearly 90% of all neck lumps. If none of these are present, look for other lesions using the list above. The following signs are helpful:	
	Fluctuation	Branchial cyst, large thyroglossal cyst and cystic hygroma often fluctuate
	Compressibility	Pharyngeal pouch empties when compressed
	Pulsation Bruit (make sure it is not a murmur transmitted from the heart)	Occur in arterial aneurysm – carotid, subclavian, axillary arteries. Also in thyrotoxicosis
	Transillumination	Occurs in cystic hygroma, some thyroglossal cysts
Examination of upper limbs	Neurological examination and examination of arterial system	Cervical rib and arterial aneurysm may produce weakness of the small muscles of the hand, trophic changes, gangrene and reduced or absent pulses
		Infection or malignancy of the upper limbs may produce a lymph node in the neck
Systematic examination	Breasts: examine carefully as indicated above for infection or malignancy CVS RS	Look for evidence of bronchial carcinoma and TB

135

Reason for examination	Sign elicited	Comment
	Abdomen: Mass, ascites, enlarged liver	Think of malignant disease in abdomen, especially from stomach
	Enlarged spleen	Consider lymphoma or leukaemia
	Testicular swelling in male	Think of tumour of testis or TB
	PR and, in women, vaginal examination	Do not forget pelvic malignancy such as carcinoma of the ovary
	CNS	Arterial aneurysms may cause neurological deficit such as weakness or sensory loss due to poor cerebral blood flow or embolism; cranial nerve damage can result from a tumour in the neck; secondary deposits in the brain can produce neurological impairment

Investigations

Many swellings in the neck can be diagnosed by history and examination alone. These include *thyroglossal cyst, branchial cyst, cervical rib, aneurysm* and *cystic hygroma. Pharyngeal pouch* can often be diagnosed clinically or at least suspected from the history. A barium swallow will be needed to determine its position, size and degree of compression of the oesophagus.

If the lump is a *submandibular salivary gland* and there is a calculus visible or palpable in the duct, investigation may be unnecessary. In some cases, an X-ray of the floor of the mouth will show a radio-opaque calculus in the gland or in the duct. This X-ray is taken by putting a small X-ray plate in the patient's mouth and taking a picture of the floor of the mouth by directing the X-ray beam from beneath the mandible. If no calculus can be identified and the clinical features are typical of obstruction of the duct, a sialogram should be requested. In this test, the orifice of the submandibular duct is cannulated and X-ray contrast injected to outline the duct and the gland. Stones obstructing the duct will be identified; changes in the gland due to duct obstruction and infection, namely dilatation of the ducts within the gland and destruction of the acini, will be seen.

The rest of the investigations described here are for the diagnosis of enlarged *lymph nodes, where the aetiology is unclear*. Lymph nodes can be recognized easily: the location in the neck, the discrete nature of the swelling, the consistency and mobility often suggest this diagnosis. It is a common mistake to proceed to biopsy in order to establish the diagnosis. While making a diagnosis is important, a poorly planned biopsy procedure may reduce the chance of curing a head and neck carcinoma which has metastasized to the cervical nodes, by encouraging further spread. It is vital to determine, wherever possible, the disease process, the source of a primary tumour and the extent of its spread. If there is any doubt the patient should be referred to an ear, nose and throat surgeon for full examination of the upper respiratory tract.

Hb: If anaemia is present, suspect a chronic infection such as TB, leukaemia or lymphoma, or carcinoma.

WCC: A grossly elevated white cell count (e.g. 40 x 10^9/l or more) should suggest a diagnosis of leukaemia, although a normal count does not exclude it. Infectious mononucleosis may sometimes give a blood picture which can be confused with leukaemia.

Blood film: The haematologist will examine the blood film if there is any suggestion of haematological disorder and will report on the morphology of the red cells, white cells, platelets, and on any abnormal cells present in the peripheral circulation.

ESR: This may be elevated in chronic infection and malignant disease. Although it is non-specific, it may be the first indication of disease.

LFTs: These may be abnormal in TB, infectious mononucleosis, leukaemia and lymphoma, and carcinoma. An abnormality may be due to infiltration of the liver.

Chest X-ray: There may be enlargement of the mediastinal lymph nodes which will show as increased opacification of the hilum of the lungs. This suggests diseases such as sarcoidosis, lymphoma (especially Hodgkin's disease), TB and carcinoma. Abnormalities of the lung fields (opacities, mass lesions, collapse, consolidation) should raise the suspicion of TB, secondary carcinoma, aspiration pneumonia due to pharyngeal pouch and primary bronchogenic carcinoma.

Barium swallow and meal: Indicated if the patient has dysphagia or if the symptoms suggest carcinoma of the stomach. Upper gastrointestinal endoscopy will be required to allow inspection and biopsy of any suspicious lesions.

Needle aspiration: This procedure should be considered next. The advantages are that it can be done without admitting the patient to hospital, and will give the diagnosis in some malignancies such as metastatic squamous carcinoma. Others, such a lymphoma, are difficult to diagnose on needle biopsy. A needle is inserted through the skin into the node, under local anaesthesia if necessary, and cells aspirated. Occasionally, a branchial cyst or tuberculous lymph node can be aspirated to provide material for culture.

Open lymph node biopsy: The following are the indications for open lymph node biopsy:

1. If lymphoma is suspected: a confident diagnosis of lymphoma cannot be made from a needle aspiration specimen; at least a core of tissue is required.

2. There is no evidence of local infection or of primary malignant tumour; systemic infection (e.g. TB, toxoplasmosis) and leukaemia should therefore be considered. Any tissue or material obtained should be sent to the laboratory for routine culture, culture for tuberculosis and for histology.

Case report

Features	Analysis
Marie Jones is 27 years old and single. She is at university doing research in biochemistry for a PhD degree. She presented to her GP during her summer holiday with a painless lump on the right side her neck, noticed 3 months before.	The commonest painless lateral neck lump at this age is a lymph node. Branchial cysts can occur but are rare. We must think of submandibular salivary gland and a preliminary examination of the neck will determine if this is a possibility. Pharyngeal pouch and an aneurysm are unlikely at this age.
She admitted to not feeling well for over 6 months and during this period her appetite had diminished and she lost 8 kg in weight. She also noticed previously easy tasks such as cleaning and cooking required more effort on her part. She gave up playing squash, which she used to enjoy. Some nights she would wake up feeling hot, shivering, and covered in sweat.	A period of illness associated with a lump in the neck should raise the possibility of chronic infection such as TB and malignancy. At this age, assuming that this nodule is a lymph node, the malignancies not to forget are lymphoma, especially Hodgkin's disease, and thyroid cancer. Think also of infectious mononucleosis (glandular fever) and other head and neck diseases.
While washing 3 months ago, she noticed a lump on the right side of her neck. It was not painful or tender, but had increased slightly in size. She did not think there were any other lumps elsewhere and had no pain.	
There were no other symptoms on systems review. In particular, she had no sore throat, cough or sputum, and as far as she knew, she had not been in contact with anyone with TB. She had no abdominal pain, jaundice or change in bowel habits, and denied urinary symptoms.	Review of symptoms is most important. It enables you to uncover disorders that may be responsible for the nodule in the neck. Malignancies in the thorax, abdomen and pelvis can sometimes present with secondaries in the neck.

Features	Analysis
She spent 2 months teaching in a mission school in East Africa 3 years ago. She was immunized against yellow fever, typhoid, cholera and hepatitis B before she left and was well throughout her stay in Africa.	The nodule may be due to a tropical infection. She had taken reasonable precautions before her trip and had no symptoms during her stay in Africa. We must not forget AIDS.
She had had no serious illness in the past. She had tonsillectomy at the age of 4 years, but no other operations.	
She did not smoke or drink alcohol. She had been on the oral contraceptive pill for 2 years.	Alcohol sometimes causes pain in a lymph node in Hodgkin's disease.
On examination she looked well and was not anaemic or jaundiced. She was apyrexial. There was no finger clubbing and no oedema.	
There was a firm nodule 2.5 cm in diameter in the anterior triangle of the neck, just anterior to the middle of the sternomastoid muscle. It felt firm, was not tender, and was fully mobile. There were no other nodules in the neck and the thyroid was not palpable. Examination of the ears, nose and throat was normal.	This nodule is almost certainly a lymph node. A normal thyroid on clinical examination does not exclude cancer. Examination of the ears, nose and throat is important to rule out disease in these areas.
The chest was clear. BP was 110/80 and pulse 80/min and regular, and heart sounds were normal. There were no palpable axillary lymph nodes.	Other node-bearing areas such as the axillae and groins must be examined to see if lymph node enlargement is confined to the neck or is present elsewhere.

There were no abnormalities on abdominal examination: the liver and spleen were not palpable. There were no abnormal inguinal nodes. Vaginal and rectal examination were normal and there were no abnormalities in the lower limbs.

The liver and spleen must be examined carefully in any patient with lymph node enlargement. The chest, abdomen and pelvis should also be examined for evidence of primary disease in these areas.

Clinical diagnosis

The most likely diagnosis is Hodgkin's disease. Her age, the nature of her systemic symptoms and the presence of a lymph node are in favour of this diagnosis. Infectious mononucleosis, though less likely, should be excluded. TB and thyroid cancer should be borne in mind.

Investigations

Hb was 11.2 g/dl; WCC 8.5x10⁹/l; ESR 120 mm in the first hour; blood film normal, no abnormal lymphocytes; Paul-Bunnel test negative.

U&Es and LFTs normal.

The Hb is low and the ESR elevated. These are non-specific but suggest current or recent illness. Note that the Paul-Bunnel test is negative 3 months after an attack of glandular fever. TB is a possibility.

Chest X-ray clear. No evidence of enlarged hilar lymph nodes.

Ultrasound of the abdomen showed normal liver, spleen, biliary tree and pancreas.

There were no enlarged para-aortic lymph nodes.

Chest X-ray and ultrasound are useful in looking for primary disease and other areas of lymph node enlargement. These conditions may be present despite the negative tests.

Ear nose and throat examination by an ENT specialist showed no abnormalities.

This must be done before the lymph node is subjected to open biopsy.

Features	Analysis
Diagnosis on lymph node biopsy Hodgkin's lymphoma. TB culture was negative.	The stage of the disease must be determined by CT scan as this is important in deciding on the mode of treatment and for determining prognosis. Lymph nodes must always be sent for culture when TB cannot be ruled out.

Chapter 9

Enlargement of, or lump in, the thyroid gland

Includes suspected hyperthyroidism and hypothyroidism

A *goitre* is any enlargement of the thyroid gland. It is a simple matter to decide whether a lump in the neck is arising from the thyroid gland: ask the patient to swallow (it often helps to give him a glass of water) and watch the lump. If the lump is in the thyroid it will ascend with swallowing. If it does not it is unlikely to be in the thyroid. The diagnosis of neck lumps outside the thyroid gland was discussed in Chapter 8.

Classification of thyroid enlargement

Congenital

(a) Cretinism

Acquired

(a) Physiological:
  (i) Diffuse enlargement at puberty, during menstruation and in pregnancy

(b) Inflammatory:
  (i) Acute thyroiditis, may be due to viral or bacterial infection
  (ii) Chronic thyroiditis; TB, Hashimoto's, Riedel's, and de Quervain's disease

(c) Thyrotoxic
  (i) Primary hyperthyroidism
  (ii) Toxic nodular goitre

(d) Hypothyroid
  (i) Myxoedema
  (ii) Drug induced
  (iii) Cretinism

(e) Simple
  (i) Solitary – cyst due to haemorrhage into a degenerative nodule
        – benign adenoma
  (ii) Multiple – nodular colloid goitre

(f) Malignant
   (i) Carcinoma – papillary
                 – follicular
                 – medullary
                 – anaplastic

Common causes of thyroid enlargement

Multinodular colloid goitre (75%), physiological goitre (6%), primary thyrotoxicosis (5%), cyst (5%), adenoma (5%)

Rare but important causes

Carcinoma, thyroiditis

Points to look for

The most common findings are as follows:

(a) Patient euthyroid

If the gland is diffusely and smoothly enlarged, the goitre is probably physiological in a pubertal person or a in woman who is pregnant or menstruating.

If a nodule is believed to be solitary on clinical grounds alone, the patient often has other nodules in the thyroid which are not palpable.

A multinodular gland is most commonly due to a nodular colloid goitre, which is frequently benign. The truly solitary nodule may be a follicular adenoma or a cyst, but there is a 15% chance of it being malignant.

(b) Patient hyperthyroid

In a young patient with a diffusely enlarged thyroid and eye signs (see text), the diagnosis is primary hyperthyroidism (Graves' disease). In older patients the gland is more often nodular and there may be atrial fibrillation or heart failure. The diagnosis is toxic nodular goitre. Malignant disease of the thyroid is almost never present in a patient who is hyperthyroid. Rarely, thyrotoxicosis may be due to a single functioning thyroid nodule. The rest of the gland is suppressed.

(c) Patient hypothyroid

Hypothyroidism may be present with Hashimoto's disease or multinodular goitre. The patient may have had previous thyroidectomy.

In primary thyroid failure the whole gland is enlarged. The enlargement is initially diffuse but later the thyroid becomes nodular.

In a baby or infant, the diagnosis is probably cretinism. This condition is rare.

The possible causes of thyroid enlargement, depending on thyroid status, are summarized below:

	Euthyroid	*Hyperthyroid*	*Hypothyroid*
Gland smoothly enlarged	Physiological	Primary hyperthyroidism	Early stages of thyroid failure
Solitary nodule	Follicular adenoma Cyst Malignancy	Functioning adenoma	Previous thyroidectomy: nodule is an underfunctioning remnant
Multinodular gland	Benign nodular colloid goitre	Nodular toxic goitre	Later stages of thyroid failure Hashimoto's disease

History

Reason for question	Question asked	Comment
Find out more about goitre. Question the patient as for any other lump	When did you first become aware of a lump in your neck? How did you discover it? Has it changed in size since then? Has there been a recent rapid increase in size? Is it painful or tender?	Diffuse enlargement of the thyroid just before periods or during pregnancy is physiological. Rapid increase may be due to haemorrhage into a cyst or to malignant change Pain occurs in thyroiditis and in a cyst into which haemorrhage has occurred
What is the goitre doing to other neck structures?	Do you have any difficulty swallowing? Have you noticed any change in your voice? Has your voice become husky? Do you get unduly short of breath or experience a choking sensation in your neck?	Large multinodular goitres and malignant tumours can cause compression or, in the case of malignancy, infiltration of the trachea or the oesophagus Recurrent laryngeal nerve paralysis is most often due to carcinoma
What is the goitre doing to the patient as a whole? i.e. is the patient hyperthyroid, hypothyroid or euthyroid?	*Symptoms of activity:* What sort of weather do you prefer? What are your nerves like? Are you nervous, irritable and easily excitable? Tell me about your sleeping pattern? Can you get to sleep easily? How many hours do you sleep for? At what time do you wake up? Do you sweat excessively?	Enquiries into metabolic state of patient. In thyrotoxicosis the patient prefers cold weather, is nervous and irritable, sleeps poorly and wakes up often; he also sweats excessively

GIT	Tell me about your appetite and your weight What are your bowel habits like? Have they changed?	In thyrotoxicosis appetite increases but weight decreases. Diarrhoea occurs in thyrotoxicosis, while constipation is more frequent in myxoedema
CVS	Are you sometimes aware of your own heartbeat (palpitations)? How fast does your heart beat? Do you get any pain in your chest? What brings it on? (Walking, eating, cold weather, going upstairs) Do you get short of breath easily when you exercise? Have you noticed any swelling of your ankles?	In thyrotoxicosis the patient gets palpitations; some have angina of effort; older patients may present with symptoms of heart failure such as orthopnoea and paroxysmal nocturnal dyspnoea and ankle oedema, but without marked metabolic disturbance
GUS	In younger woman: has there been a change in your periods? How frequently do you have a period, and how much blood do you lose?	In thyrotoxicosis the patient may develop amenorrhoea or scanty irregular periods
Attempt to find a cause for the thyroid enlargement	Do you come from an area where goitres (lumps in the thyroid) are common? What medicines are you taking?	Multinodular goitres are common in people from areas where goitres are endemic Certain drugs such as phenylbutazone and resorcinol (now rarely used) suppress thyroid activity. Antithyroid drugs such as carbimazole and propylthiouracil can cause hypothyroidism and goitre

Reason for question	Question asked	Comment
	In a woman, is swelling related to periods? If pregnant, has it come up since becoming pregnant?	Physiological goitre
ROS	Many of the systems will already have been enquired into. Finish enquiry into RS, CVS, CNS, GUS, GIT	
PMH	Previous history of thyroid disease, thyroid operation or treatment with radioactive iodine	
FH	Are there any other members of your family with thyroid disease?	Medullary carcinoma (a rare condition) may be familial. Goitres in a family may also be due to living in an endemic area
SH, DRUGS, ALLERGIES	Some of the points have been covered above	

Examination

Reason for examination	Sign elicited	Comment
General well-being	Look for general signs of malignancy. They include cachexia, anaemia and jaundice.	

Any general signs of hypo- or hyperthyroidism	In general the hyperthyroid patient, more often female, is thin, nervous and fidgety, and has sweaty warm skin. She has a fine tremor of the outstretched hand. The hypothyroid patient (also usually female), on the other hand, is obese, depressed and moves about sluggishly. Her skin is cold and dry. Remember, however, that these signs occur in more severe cases and may be absent in those with mild disease. In rare cases of hypherthyroidism, the signs are the opposite to those stated above.	
	Skin changes of thyroid disease	Coarse dry skin and sparse hair in myxoedema; pretibial myxoedema (oedematous swellings above lateral maleoli in thyrotoxicosis)
	Pubertal. If woman of child bearing age, is she pregnant?	Consider physiological goitre if the goitre is diffusely enlarged and soft
Any eye signs of thyrotoxicosis?	Exophthalmos Lid retraction/ lid lag Ophthalmoplegia	Normally the sclera is not visible below the lower border of the iris. In thyrotoxicosis the eyeballs bulge forwards, and the voluntary and involuntary muscles associated with eye movements may be weak in more severe cases of eye disease
NECK: systematic examination most important	*Inspection:* Where is the swelling? In one or other lobe of the thyroid or is the whole gland affected? Watch the swelling as the patient swallows	
	Does it move when the patient sticks the tongue out?	Exclude thyroglossal cyst

149

Reason for examination	Sign elicited	Comment
	Any other swellings such as lymph nodes?	Think of malignancy
	Palpation: Palpate the thyroid from behind; answer same questions as on inspection. In addition:	
	Can you get below the gland?	Retrosternal extension is more likely with multinodular goitre and occasionally with carcinoma
	If lymph node found, where exactly is it in the neck?	Metastatic nodes from thyroid cancer are often found behind the medial part of the lower third of the sternomastoid muscle
	Is the gland diffusely enlarged and smooth?	As in primary hyperthyroidism
	Is it woody hard?	As in chronic thyroiditis
	Is it tender?	As in acute thyroiditis
	Is the gland diffusely enlarged and nodular?	As in multinodular goitre
	Is there only one nodule, and is the rest of the gland normal?	This is a clinically solitary nodule. Most often there are other nodules which are not easily palpable, in which case the patient has a multinodular goitre. The significance of the clinically solitary nodule is that it can be malignant

Are there features of malignancy, such as a fixed nodule, or hoarse voice suggesting recurrent laryngeal nerve paralysis?

Feel the trachea: is it central or is it deviated? — The commonest cause of tracheal deviation is a multinodular goitre, and occasionally cancer

Percussion: percuss over the lower part of the gland to determine whether retrosternal extension is present — This is not an easy examination for students

Auscultation: is there a bruit present? — Suggesting thyrotoxicosis

RS

Any signs of airways obstruction? — Due to tracheal compression

Any signs of lung collapse or consolidation? — Suggesting secondary carcinoma

CVS

Blood pressure — Systolic hypertension sometimes present in hyperthyroidism

Pulse rate and rhythm — Tachycardia in hyperthyroidism, even when the patient is asleep. Atrial fibrillation commoner in older patients with hyperthyroidism

JVP, apex beat, cardiac thrills, murmurs, crackles — In older patients with hyperthyroidism, heart failure is sometimes a presenting feature. There may be a systolic murmur due to increased blood flow

151

Reason for examination	Sign elicited	Comment
CNS	Test muscle power and elicit tendon reflexes	Proximal myopathy is present in a large proportion of hyperthyroid patients; tendon reflexes are increased Tendon reflexes are sluggish in hypothyroidism
ABDOMEN		
SKELETAL SYSTEM		Thyroid cancer can spread to bone

Investigations

First confirm thyroid status

Most laboratories first measure the level of thyroid stimulating hormone (TSH) in blood. A normal value can be accepted as evidence that the patient is euthyroid. If the TSH level is abnormal, the level of free thyroxine (T_4) or triiodothyronine (T_3) is measured. A low TSH and high T_3 confirm hyperthyroidism, and a high TSH and low T_4 hypothyroidism. A low TSH may sometimes give the false impression of hyperthyroidism in patients whose thyroid is not overactive.

Patient euthyroid

Most patients presenting with a goitre are euthyroid.
Whole gland enlarged and smooth – physiological goitre. No further tests are required.
Whole gland enlarged and nodular, or multiple nodules – multinodular goitre. This is usually benign, but if there is doubt about malignancy, fine needle

aspiration cytology should be done. Also, chest and thoracic inlet X-rays are sometimes done to detect tracheal compression and large retrosternal extension.

Single nodule – 10–15% risk of malignancy. Fine needle aspiration is important. An ultrasound scan of the thyroid will tell whether the lump is wholly cystic, partly cystic or entirely solid. Solid lumps are more likely to be malignant than cystic ones, which are very rarely so. Ultrasound will also show the presence of other (impalpable) nodules of a multinodular goitre.

Other tests: iodine scan to determine whether the lump is cold or hot. A cold nodule has a 10–15% risk of malignancy.

Malignancy proved on biopsy

FBC and chest X-ray are performed before an operation; also an ENT surgeon should be asked to check the vocal cords.

Interpretation of tests in patients with thyroid swelling

Hb and ESR: Anaemia and raised ESR may be due to carcinoma. Anaemia may be present in myxoedema.

LFTs: Abnormal LFTs may be due to secondary carcinoma in the liver. In such a case there will be obvious evidence of a primary tumour, often with lymph node involvement.

ECG: This will show tachycardia in thyrotoxicosis; atrial fibrillation may be present. In myxoedema there is sinus bradycardia and low voltage waves.

X-rays of chest, neck and thoracic inlet: These may reveal a soft tissue swelling in the neck. The position of the trachea should be noted and the presence of compression or of deviation should be determined. Retrosternal extension will be seen on the inlet and chest films. The lung fields should be inspected for evidence of secondary carcinoma or heart failure.

Tests of thyroid status: These are discussed above.

Thyroid autoantibodies: These are sometimes present in Grave's disease and commonly in chronic thyroiditis (Hashimoto's disease).

Isotope scanning of the thyroid: This is done by administering a small dose of a radioactive substance which is taken up by the thyroid gland. The isotopes commonly used are iodine and technetium. The scan gives a visual image of the thyroid: functioning thyroid cells take up the isotope, and non-functioning areas do not. A cold nodule is one which does not take up isotope while the surrounding thyroid does, and a hot nodule is one which takes up isotope when the rest of the thyroid does not. If a nodule is found to be solitary clinically and is cold on scan, the risk of its being malignant is nearly 15%.

Thyroid ultrasound scan: This is especially useful in determining whether a single nodule is indeed solitary or whether the gland is, in fact, multinodular. Small nodules which are often impalpable will show on the scan. It will also determine whether the nodule is solid or cystic: a cystic nodule is either a simple cyst or a colloid cyst. A solid nodule may be an adenoma or carcinoma.

Fine needle aspiration cytology of the thyroid: In this technique cells are aspirated from the thyroid gland and sent for cytology. In expert hands, it is very useful for diagnosing thyroid lumps. Follicular adenomas are extremely difficult to distinguish from carcinomas on cytological grounds. A negative result must not be accepted as evidence that there is no malignancy.

Case report

Features	Analysis
Fatma Ahmed is a 36-year-old housewife. She lives with her husband and their two young children. They are from Pakistan. Two weeks before she went to see her GP, a friend of the family remarked that she had a lump in her neck. She had not been aware of this swelling.	Note the patient's age and sex. Thyroid swellings are common at this age, and it is not unusual for the lump to be discovered by someone else.
The lump was on the left side of her neck and was not painful or tender. She did not notice any change in her voice, difficulty in swallowing or shortness of breath.	Malignant swellings of the thyroid are often painless, but most thyroid lumps are benign. There are no symptoms of compression or infiltration of neck structures.

Detailed enquiry about her thyroid status did not suggest any symptoms of overactivity or underactivity of the thyroid, and there were no significant symptoms on systems review.

Most patients with thyroid swellings are euthyroid. There are no symptoms to suggest malignancy.

She admitted that goitres were common in the area of Pakistan from which they came and where they lived until she was aged 20, but no members of her immediate family were known to have goitres. She was not taking any regular medications and had not had any serious illnesses or operations.

Goitres are probably endemic in her town of origin, but there is no reason to suspect that her thyroid swelling is endemic in origin. She was not on any possibly goitrogenic drugs and had had no thyroid operations.

On examination she looked well though obese. She was not anaemic or jaundiced.
There were no general signs of thyroid overactivity or underactivity. The eyes and skin were normal.

Always look for signs of altered thyroid status.

There was a swelling 3.5 cm in diameter on the left side of her neck below the level of the thyroid cartilage and partly under cover of the sternomastoid muscle. It was non-tender and mobile. It was soft and globular in shape, and moved up and then down when she swallowed. The lower border of this mass was easily felt when it moved upwards on swallowing. The rest of the thyroid was not palpable. There were no lymph nodes in the neck or axillae.
The trachea was central and both common carotid pulses were easily felt. There were no bruits over the gland.

This is a clinically solitary nodule. In many cases, it is a dominant nodule in a multinodular goitre; the other nodules are not easily palpable. The significance is the possibility of malignancy. There is no sign of retrosternal extension and no tracheal deviation.

155

Features	Analysis
BP was 115/75, pulse 84/min, regular and of good volume. Examination of the lungs and heart revealed no abnormalities. All peripheral pulses were normal.	Complete systemic examination is important to confirm that the patient is euthyroid and has no other disease.
The abdomen, groins and lower limbs were normal. Neurological examination was normal.	

Clinical diagnosis
This patient presented with a clinically solitary nodule. She may have a multinodular non-toxic goitre for reasons discussed above. However, if this nodule proves to be solitary, it may be a cyst or a benign follicular adenoma. There is, however, a 15% chance of malignancy.

Investigations

Fine needle aspiration of the nodule showed a solid mass. Cytology showed a follicular neoplasm. It was not possible to determine from cytology whether this was benign or malignant.	As mentioned above, it is often difficult to distinguish a follicular adenoma from a follicular carcinoma from cytology alone.

Thyroid function tests were normal. Ultrasound of the thyroid showed a solitary, solid 3.5 cm mass in the lower pole of the left lobe of the thyroid. A technetium scan showed this to be a cold nodule, increasing further the possibility of malignancy. Chest X-ray was normal.

Final diagnosis
She underwent neck exploration and left thyroid lobectomy. Frozen section examination and later paraffin sections showed a benign follicular adenoma of the thyroid.

Chapter 10

Lump in the breast

Over 96% of lumps in the breast are benign, but a good history and examination are essential to ensure that carcinoma is not missed.

Causes of lumps in the breast (* indicates those lumps most commonly found in practice or most important)

(a) Benign tumours:
  (i) Fibroadenoma*
  (ii) Duct papilloma
  (iii) Lipoma
  (iv) Cyst: galactocele
         single cyst in fibroadenosis*
  (v) Fibroadenosis*
  (vi) Abscess
  (vii) Fat necrosis
(b) Malignant tumours:
  (i) Carcinoma*
  (ii) Sarcoma

Common causes

Fibroadenosis (80%), single cyst in fibroadenosis (8%), fibroadenoma (5%), carcinoma (1–2%).

Points to look for

Fibroadenosis

The patient with fibroadenosis is usually in her thirties or early forties. The main feature is cyclical pain, usually occurring in the week or so before periods, and lessening with periods. In many patients the pain is not cyclical. The pain may be localized over the area of the lump or it may be in the whole breast. The breast is generally lumpy on examination and the swelling with which she presents may be merely a dominant nodule in a nodular breast. There is often tenderness in the nodular parts of the breast. One of these nodules may be a cyst.

Fibroadenoma

The patient with fibroadenoma is usually in her twenties (younger than the patient with fibroadenosis). She presents with a painless lump. Examination reveals a discrete, fully circumscribed, firm swelling which is mobile. This lesion is sometimes referred to as a 'breast mouse' because of this mobility. While such characteristics make such a lump most likely to be a fibroadenoma, carcinoma cannot be absolutely excluded.

Carcinoma

Breast carcinoma can present at any age, but is often seen in women aged 40 and over. The patient commonly presents with a painless lump. The presence of pain does not exclude a carcinoma; pain from breast cancer is sometimes described as 'pricking'. Obvious signs of malignancy such as ulceration, fungation, peau d'orange and eczema of the nipple are not common. The lump is firm and poorly circumscribed, and its mobility is reduced.

At the end of the examination you should be able to place the patient in one of three management categories: (a) almost certainly benign, (b) almost certainly malignant, and (c) not sure. Further investigations depend on this provisional categorization and on the patient's age. Thus a patient in category (a) who is in her twenties, if otherwise fit, need only have a haemoglobin estimation (if at all) and then excision of the lump. Most of the other tests outlined below are needed only in patients in categories (b) and (c).

History

Reason for question	Question asked	Comment
Find out more about the lump and its cause	Please show me exactly where the lump is When did you first discover the lump? What brought your attention to this lump?	Sometimes there may be a history of trauma, in which case the diagnosis is likely to be fat

necrosis. This occurs only if trauma is enough to cause bruising; the condition is virtually confined to the obese breast. Many patients with cancer will say that the lump appeared after injury. The trauma often is incidental and draws the patient's attention to the lump

Do you examine your breasts regularly?	Women are advised to examine their own breasts regularly in the hope that any lumps will be discovered earlier
Has the lump changed in size since it was first discovered?	A rapidly enlarging lump should arouse suspicion of cancer
If she still has periods: Is there any relationship between the appearance of this lump and your periods?	If the lump appears in the week before a period and regresses after, it is often due to fibroadenosis. The 'lump' referred to by the patient is an increase in the nodularity of the breast
Is the lump painful or does it hurt when you touch it?	The pain of fibroadenosis is sometimes (but not always) cyclical. Pain may be due to an abscess. Some patients with carcinoma describe a pricking pain. Most carcinomas and fibroadenomas are painless

Reason for question	Question asked	Comment
Changes at the nipple	Any discharge from your nipple? If so, what colour is it?	Bloody discharge is due to carcinoma or duct papilloma. An excess of milky discharge is referred to as galactorrhoea. Greeny discharge occurs in fibroadenosis and duct ectasia
	If nipple discharge present: Is the discharge always from the same place on the nipple or from different sites?	A bloody discharge from the same location is due to either intraduct papilloma or carcinoma
	Have you noticed a rash or redness around the nipple?	An intraduct carcinoma often presents with eczema of the nipple, and the condition is known as Paget's disease of the breast
	Has there been any recent change in your weight? How do you feel in yourself?	Possibility of carcinoma, but note that most women presenting with breast carcinoma for the first time are well
ROS	GIT	
	RS: cough, sputum, haemoptysis, pleuritic chest pain, dyspnoea?	Chest symptoms should be sought, as they may point to secondary deposits in the lungs from breast cancer
	CVS	
	CNS: full nervous system enquiry.	Secondaries can occur in the brain

	GUS: When was menarche established? Is the patient pre- peri- or post-menopausal?	The prognosis and the treatment of breast cancer depend on the menopausal status of the woman
	How many pregnancies has she had? How many live births? Were any children breast fed? If yes, for how long each?	Multiparous women who have breast fed are less likely than nulliparous women to have breast cancer
	SKELETAL: Any pain in any bones? Has she had any bone fractures after trivial injury?	Secondary deposits in bone cause pain and can produce pathological fractures
PMH	Any history of breast disease or breast operations? Have you had radiation treatment to the breast in the past?	Enquire about previous treatment for breast cancer or for benign breast disease
FH	Does anyone in the family suffer from breast disease?	10–15% of patients with breast cancer have a family history of the disease. A family history is significant for an individual if mother and/or sister had breast cancer premenopausally
SH		

161

Reason for question	Question asked	Comment
DRUGS	*Oral contraceptive pill*	There is, however, no proven link between the pill and breast cancer, but women on the pill are believed to be more liable to develop benign breast disease
ALLERGIES		

Examination

Reason for examination	Sign elicited	Comment
General well-being; signs of spread of breast cancer	A patient with advanced breast cancer may be ill, thin, anaemic and jaundiced. Such patients are rare nowadays. Examine for cervical and supraclavicular lymph node enlargement now. The axilla is examined with the breast below. In practice, many of the examinations below looking for signs of secondary tumour are only carried out in those who are likely or have been proved to have malignancy.	
BREASTS	Always examine both breasts carefully and compare affected with normal breast.	
Is there a lump or change that suggests malignancy?	*Inspection:* Compare the two breasts	The two breasts are often unequal but one breast may be larger because of carcinoma or phyllodes tumour (the so-called 'giant fibroadenoma')

Are the breast contours normal and symmetrical?	An area of asymmetry may be the site of carcinoma
Any skin dimpling?	
Any peau d'orange?	This is oedema of the skin and gives the appearance of an orange peel, hence the name
Inspect the skin all over the breast: is there any rash, discoloration, or redness?	A rash may be due to eczema or Paget's disease; redness may be due to infection
Is there any ulceration?	Ulceration most often due to fungating carcinoma. This is rare
Now look carefully at the nipples and the areola: are the two nipples at the same level?	A carcinoma in one breast may pull the nipple upwards
Is there inversion of one or of both nipples? If yes, is it recent?	Inversion, especially if recent, should alert you to the possibility of carcinoma
Ask the patient to bend forwards and see if both breasts fall freely off the chest wall	Failure of the breast to fall may be because it is tethered by carcinoma
Inspect the arms: is one arm obviously swollen?	Swelling may be due to lymphoedema caused by carcinoma
Ask the patient to raise her arms well above her head: is there now any puckering or swelling which was not obvious when the arm was by the side?	This may reveal the position of a carcinoma

Reason for examination	Sign elicited	Comment
If a lump is present, is it benign or malignant on palpation?	Palpation: Examine both breasts fully Is there a lump? If there is, determine its characteristics as described in the Introduction	Reduced mobility is because the lump is tethered to the underlying pectoral muscle by tumour
	Palpate the axilla carefully and systematically. If any lump is there, what are its characteristics?	Lymph nodes in the presence of a lump in the breast are highly likely to contain secondary carcinoma
	Examine the arms: any lymphoedema or dilated veins?	Suggesting obstruction by malignant tissue
RS	Examine for signs of collapse, consolidation and pleural effusion	These suggest secondary carcinoma in the lungs
CVS		
CNS		Neurological abnormalities can occur because of direct damage to neural tissue by tumour (for instance hemiparesis due to brain secondary) or indirectly as a result of carcinomatous neuropathy. There may be papilloedema due to raised intracranial pressure. All of these are uncommon nowadays

ABDOMEN	The main reason for examining the abdomen in a patient with a breast lump, especially one with features suggestive of malignancy, is to determine whether or not secondaries are present. Signs that should raise suspicion are: ascites, mass, enlarged liver with irregular edge and enlarged inguinal lymph nodes.
SKELETAL SYSTEM	Examine for evidence of bone secondaries by eliciting bone tenderness and reduced movement in spine and other joints.

Investigations

The investigations performed depend on the findings on history and examination.

Nodular area, no discrete nodule

The diagnosis is probably fibroadenosis. Mammography or xeroradiography (if available) is helpful in women over the age of 35. Below this age, the breasts are usually too radiodense to show small abnormalities clearly. Ultrasound is used instead of mammography in women under the age of 35. If there are features of malignancy, the suspicious area is biopsied.

Discrete lump

Fine needle aspiration of mass for cytological examination. If there is doubt, open biopsy is done. Needle aspiration is important in the management of breast cysts. If the cyst disappears and does not recur, and fluid does not contain malignant cells on cytological examination, no further action is needed.

Malignancy confirmed by cytology of aspirated material or histology of excised tissue

Full blood count, liver function tests, chest X-ray, ultrasound of the liver.

Additional tests: isotope scanning of the liver and bones and brain CT scan.

Interpretation of tests in patients with breast lumps

Blood tests and X-rays are indicated only if carcinoma is confirmed. They are of little value if the lump is benign.

Hb: There may be anaemia in a patient with malignancy, but even with carcinoma the haemoglobin is often normal.

LFTs: If abnormal, may be due to secondary carcinoma in the liver.

Chest X-ray: Is of value if carcinoma is present. It may show secondaries in the lungs and in the ribs.

Fine needle aspiration cytology (FNAC): Aspiration is carried out with a 21 or 23 gauge needle attached to a syringe. The needle is inserted through the skin into the abnormal area and material obtained by withdrawing the plunger. Multiple passes of the needle are often necessary to loosen cells and increase the volume of aspirate. The plunger is released before the needle is withdrawn from the lesion to ensure the aspirate does not get sucked into the syringe. The material is spread thinly on microscope slides, fixed and sent to the laboratory for staining and cytological examination.

FNAC is done if there is a discrete lump or a suspicious area. Its advantage is that it may enable a diagnosis of carcinoma to be made without open biopsy. The precise operation to be undertaken can then be discussed with the patient beforehand. Negative cytology does not exclude carcinoma.

If fluid is aspirated it should be sent for cytology; so too should discharge from the nipple.

Mammography or xeroradiography: Provides a soft tissue image of the breast. Xeroradiography gives better images than mammography but involves a greater dose of radiation to the breasts. In many clinics these tests are indicated mainly in those women who present with pain in the breast or other symptoms, in whom a discrete lump cannot be palpated, or in whom the breasts are nodular. They are also used as screening tests in women without symptoms, but the dose of radiation given must be taken into account.

Ultrasound of the breast: Ultrasound allows abnormalities in the breast to be converted into images.

Cysts are transparent and other benign lesions usually have well defined edges but cancers on the other hand have poorly defined outlines.

Triple assessment: This is the combination of clinical examination, imaging (ultrasound for women under the age of 35 and mammography for those over 35) and FNAC. This combination has an accuracy of nearly 99% in diagnosing malignancy.

Ultrasound scanning of the liver and isotope scanning of bones: These are performed if indicated in those with proved malignancy, for example if liver function tests are abnormal or if there is bone pain.

Brain CT scan: Is indicated if there are neurological symptoms or signs.

Case report

Features	Analysis
Joanne Taylor is a 25-year-old staff nurse. She is married and has one daughter. She saw her GP because of a lump she had found in her right breast 4 months ago.	Malignancy can present at any age, but as stated above, it is commoner over the age of 40.
She did not do regular breast self examination and noticed this lump accidentally while having a shower. She had been well in herself. The lump was painless and did not change during her menstrual cycle. It did not increase in size significantly over the following 4 months. There was no history of trauma to the breast and she did not have a nipple discharge.	Fibroadenoma and carcinoma can present as a painless lump in the breast and can both be present without nipple discharge.

Features	*Analysis*
Her menarche was at the age of 14 and she was married at the age of 22. She had her daughter one year later and breast fed for 3 months. She started taking the oral contraceptive pill after delivery and was on it at the time she was seen for this breast lump. Her periods were always regular.	There is no evidence that the pill increases the risk of breast cancer.
Systems review did not reveal any significant symptoms. Her appetite was good, she had not lost weight and denied bone pain. She had no cough or sputum.	Systems review is important in the search for other diseases and evidence of metastases from possible breast cancer.
She had appendicectomy at the age of 8 but had not had any other illnesses or operations. Apart from the oral contraceptive pill, she was not on any regular medication.	
On examination she was well and had no anaemia or jaundice. There were no abnormalities on examination of her head and neck. Her BP was 115/70 and pulse 72/min and regular. Her chest was clear and heart normal.	
There was a firm, spherical, well circumscribed, non-tender lump 3 cm in diameter in the upper outer quadrant of her right breast. There was no overlying skin abnormality and this lump was fully mobile and not attached to skin or to deep tissues. The rest of the right breast, the whole of the left breast and both axillae were normal.	These are the features of a benign lump and are typical of fibroadenoma, but histological confirmation is important. However, some authorities believe that most fibroadenomas diagnosed by clinical examination, USG and FNAC do not need to be excised, as the risk of malignancy is insignificant.

There were no abnormalities on abdominal examination. The
  liver and spleen were not palpable and there were no
  masses or ascites.

The rest of the examination did not show any abnormalities.

Clinical diagnosis
The clinical characteristics of this lump are those of fibroadenoma (see above). Fibroadenoma is common at this age but
  some believe histological confirmation is mandatory bearing in mind that malignancy cannot be completely ruled out.

Investigation
Fine needle aspiration showed the lump to be solid and
  cytology revealed benign cells.

Final diagnosis
The lump was excised and sent for histology. It was a
  fibroadenoma.

Chapter 11

Suspected renal tract pain

Often it is possible to ascribe pain to the kidneys or urinary tract simply from its description. Occasionally, however, the pain is atypical in its presentation and distribution, and an origin from the urinary tract will become apparent only after investigation. The patient may present to the emergency department if the pain is severe, but in some cases he attends an outpatient clinic if his pain is not severe but recurrent.

There are two classic types of renal pain: (a) fixed renal pain and (b) renal colic.

(a) Fixed renal pain

The pain is felt in the 'renal' angle, in the loin between the twelfth rib and the lateral edge of the spine, and it is constant. It may be localized in the hypochondrium, and, if on the right, it should be distinguished from other causes of pain in this area, notably gall bladder disease. Fixed renal pain is due to inflammation of the kidney or to obstruction above the pelviureteric junction.

(b) Renal and ureteric colic

Colic is defined as pain which occurs in spasms separated by pain-free intervals. Renal or ureteric pain is strictly not colic, but this expression has now found widespread usage. The pain is severe and is almost constant, but frequent exacerbations occur. It starts in the renal angle and, when severe, radiates to the iliac fossa, groin and perineum. In men radiation is to the testis or the tip of the penis, and in women to the labia. It is not possible to locate the site of the obstructing lesion from the history.

Strangury

Another, less common, type of urinary tract pain is strangury, which is an urgent and painful desire to pass urine. The pain is located in the suprapubic area and, when severe, radiates to the tip of the penis in the male and the labia in the female.

Causes of urinary tract pain (commoner causes marked *)

(a) Kidney:
  (i) Renal calculus.*
  (ii) Blood clot passing down from the kidney, for instance after injury or operation and from carcinoma.*
  (iii) Hydronephrosis, for example due to pelvi-ureteric obstruction.*
  (iv) Renal carcinoma, without the passage of blood clot.
  (v) Infection such as pyelonephritis* or rarely tuberculosis.

(b) Ureter:
  (i) Stone in the ureter.*
  (ii) Blood clot in the ureter.
  (iii) Obstruction by tuberculosis or retroperitoneal tumour.
  (iv) Stricture following injury or operation in the area of the ureter.

(c) Bladder:
  (i) Stone in the bladder.
  (ii) Foreign body in the bladder.
  (iii) Blood clot in the bladder, for example due to a bladder tumour or following operation or injury.*
  (iv) Infection or inflammation of an adjacent organ such as appendix and Fallopian tube.*

Commoner causes

Urinary tract infection (65%), ureteric calculus (25%), trauma to the urinary tract (3%), renal calculus (3%), passage of blood clot (2%).

Points to look for

Stones are a common cause of urinary pain. The exact nature of the pain and associated symptoms depend on the site of the stone. Many stones in the kidney do not produce symptoms. If a stone obstructs a calyx or the renal pelvis, it causes chronic or recurrent renal angle pain. Tenderness may be elicited in the renal angle in an attack.

During its passage through the ureter, a stone causes ureteric colic which is often recurrent. However, if a stone impacts in the ureter, it causes acute and severe unilateral ureteric colic. Chronic incomplete obstruction of the urinary tract results in hydronephrosis which may be asymptomatic; often the patient suffers from recurrent or constant loin pain. Hydronephrosis can also result from stricture or cancer in the ureter or bladder. The kidney is often enlarged and may be tender.

When a stone enters the bladder there is usually no pain. A bladder stone rarely enters the urethra; if it does, the patient gets pain on micturition. He may pass the stone or gravel in the urine.

The pain from obstructing urinary calculi is made worse by a large fluid intake, which increases distension of the urinary tract.

Stones are liable to cause urinary infection. Those in the kidney and ureter cause pyelonephritis or sometimes a perinephric abscess. The patient presents with fever and rigors, vomiting and loin pain or ureteric colic. Bladder stones cause urinary frequency and pain on micturition or 'pis-en-deux'. Urinary tract infection from other causes produces the same symptoms.

Stones cause haematuria (see next chapter). Haematuria must always be investigated to avoid missing malignancy. Renal failure can occur if both kidneys or ureters are obstructed simultaneously, or where a single functioning kidney is blocked.

Tuberculosis is not as rare as may be thought. It must be considered in an Asian patient, in a patient who has been unwell, lost weight and has night sweats. Many of the features are similar to those of carcinoma.

History

If the patient presents as an emergency, first take a quick history from which it will often be apparent that the pain is of urinary tract origin. It is common practice to confirm haematuria before a strong analgesic is given. The patient should then be given an adequate dose of a strong analgesic parenterally, for instance, pethidine 100 mg intramuscularly. Diclofenac has been shown to be equally effective. Some doctors also add an antispasmodic agent such as hyoscine butylbromide (Buscopan) 10 mg i.m. A more detailed history can then be taken from the patient once the analgesic has taken effect.

Remember that in an attempt to obtain opiate injections, some drug addicts may feign 'ureteric colic' and can even deliberately add blood to their urine to produce 'haematuria'.

Reason for question	Question asked	Comment
Find out much more about the pain	See scheme for enquiry into pain	Be sure that this is true renal tract pain. Pain from some diseases may mimic renal pain. They include cholecystitis, pancreatitis, appendicitis, salpingitis and ectopic pregnancy. Systems review should be thorough
Associated symptoms	Nausea and vomiting	These are commonly associated with renal tract pain as well as pain from other sources
	Fever and rigors	May be due to urinary infection
	Malaise, weight loss and anorexia	Suspect malignancy or uraemia if these symptoms are present
Other urinary symptoms	Frequency of micturition Urgency Nocturia Hesitancy	The presence of other urinary symptoms helps to localize the disease to the urinary tract but does not exclude pathology elsewhere. For instance, there may be severe urinary tract symptoms in patients with acute appendicitis

Reason for question	Question asked	Comment
	Haematuria	This should alert one to the possibility of malignancy but is often due to other causes (see next chapter on haematuria)
REVIEW OF SYSTEMS	*GENITAL SYSTEM: discharge per urethram; menstruation in women*	Pelvic inflammatory disease in women can produce urinary symptoms. Pelvic malignancies can obstruct the ureter
	RS: CNS: GIT:	Think of spread of renal carcinoma to the lungs or the brain. Note also that uraemia from any cause can produce CNS symptoms such as blurring of vision, muscle weakness and confusion; RS symptoms such as pleuritic chest pain and dyspnoea; and GIT symptoms such as nausea and vomiting
	CVS:	Renal artery stenosis, causing diminished blood flow to the kidney, results in hypertension
PMH	History of TB, previous renal stones, recent injury, instrumentation such as cystoscopy and urethral catheterization, pelvic operations	
FH		Urinary tract calculi may be familial

SH	Take an occupational history if haematuria present. All jobs done, especially in the chemical and rubber industry	Always take an occupational history where there is a possibility of bladder carcinoma. Smoking is an important risk factor for bladder carcinoma
	Handling aniline dyes	
	Smoking	
	Race and period abroad	Origin from northern and some other parts of Africa (especially Egypt) where schistosomiasis is common is important if bladder cancer suspected. Also bear in mind the possibility of TB in those from Asia or Africa
DRUGS, ALLERGIES		

Examination

Reason for examination	Sign elicited	Comment
How is the renal disease affecting the patient?	If the patient is ill and pyrexial, think of infection such as pyonephrosis, pyelonephritis or septicaemia.	
	A patient suffering from uraemia will also look unwell. Adequate analgesia is important in a patient in pain.	
	Look for signs of dehydration which may be present in a patient who has been vomiting and has uraemia.	
	Shock following injury or operation suggests bleeding.	
	Consider tuberculosis in malnourished patients or those with lymphadenopathy.	

Reason for examination	Sign elicited	Comment
Any signs of uraemia?	Drowsy or confused? Pale? Restless, twitching?	
RS	Rate and character of respiration	In metabolic acidosis, due for example to renal failure, respiratory rate is high and respirations are laboured
	Signs of collapse, consolidation or pleural effusion	Suggesting secondary deposits in lungs
CVS	Listen for bruit in the abdomen (lateral to the umbilicus)	Hypertension can occur in unilateral renal disease. A bruit can sometimes be heard over a stenosed renal artery
CNS	Any focal or generalized CNS signs?	Suggesting secondary carcinoma or uraemia
ABDOMEN	Scars from previous urinary and other operations. Distended?	Ascites from TB or secondary carcinoma Distended bladder may cause distension of the lower abdomen

Tenderness (especially in renal angle)	From renal tract infection or trauma
Masses	Tumour deposits, TB
Pulsatile mass	Ruptured abdominal aortic aneurysm in the older patient. This can be confused for a full bladder and the pain attributed to renal colic
Liver enlarged	Consider secondary deposits
Kidney enlarged	Think of carcinoma, hydronephrosis, TB
Bladder distended?	May be obstructed by stone or tumour
Examine genitalia for carcinoma, tuberculosis (lump in scrotum), or discharge	
Oedema of the legs	Lymphoedema may be due to obstruction of lymphatics by malignant lymph nodes; pitting oedema due to obstruction of major veins
PR: feel for prostate in men. In both sexes determine whether there are any pelvic masses	

Investigations

Urine examination: Look at the urine. Does it look cloudy or blood stained? Is there gravel or other sediment?

Urinalysis: Blood may be present and if in large quantities will be visible macroscopically. It may be due to carcinoma, stones, tuberculosis and other infections. Protein may also be present in the urine.

Urine microscopy and culture: Note the number of white cells per field, the presence of casts, of organisms and of crystalline materials. If organisms are cultured they will be identified and where indicated their bacterial sensitivities will be determined.

Pus cells in the urine: The absence of organisms (*sterile pyuria*) should alert one to TB, especially if the urine is acid. If TB is suspected, three early morning specimens of urine should be sent for special culture.

Urine cytology: A random specimen of urine is collected and sent to the laboratory. This is centrifuged and the deposit prepared for cytological examination. If malignant cells are seen, their origin in the urinary tract can be sought by other tests such as IVU and cystoscopy and ultrasound of the urinary tract.

Chemical analysis of urinary stones: Any stones retrieved from the urine should be sent for chemical analysis to determine their composition. Further advice to the patient may depend on the result of this analysis.

Hb: Anaemia may be due to uraemia or malignancy.

WCC: This may be raised when infection is present.

ESR or CRP: These may be raised if there is tumour, bacterial infection or TB.

Urea, electrolytes and creatinine: These are useful tests of renal function.

X-ray of chest: The chest X-ray may show secondary tumour or TB. It is done only if these conditions are found or are strongly suspected.

Plain X-ray of the abdomen: Showing the kidneys, ureters and bladder (KUB) is important. Look carefully at the kidney size and position. Look for opacities which may be calculi in the kidneys, ureters and bladder. Is the bladder distended?

Serum calcium and albumin: The calcium level should be corrected for an albumin of 40 mmol/l. If hypercalcaemia is found, three consecutive fasting levels should be measured, the blood having been taken without a tourniquet. Causes of hypercalcaemia such as secondary carcinoma should first be excluded before investigation is started for primary hyperparathyroidism.

Ultrasound of the kidneys: This is a very useful test, it is non-invasive, and requires no special preparation. It will demonstrate space occupying lesions in the kidneys such as tumours and cysts. It will also determine whether hydronephrosis is present.

IVU: This will show calculi in the urinary tract, space occupying lesions such as tumours, obstructions causing hydronephrosis, and the effects of long-standing infection of the urinary tract.

Further investigations may or may not be required depending on the results of the above investigations.

If a urinary calculus is found, full metabolic tests should be done to determine any underlying cause. A 24-hour specimen of urine should be sent for calcium, phosphate, urate and oxalate excretion.

Cystoscopy is mandatory if haematuria has occurred.

Further tests to determine whether there is a tumour are discussed in the next chapter on haematuria.

Case report

Features	Analysis
Jan Haynes is a 34-year-old medical representative for a large pharmaceutical company. She is separated from her husband and lives alone in a flat. She presented to the emergency department with a 5-hour history of pain in the right loin.	Several disorders immediately come to mind to account for pain in the right loin in a 34-year-old woman. The word 'loin' usually makes students think of renal diseases, but keep an open mind.
She admitted to having three similar but much milder episodes of pain in the last 2 years. Each episode lasted about an hour or two and subsided completely.	A number of diseases cause recurrent pain. Among them are gall stones, renal stones and infections, and certain gynaecological disorders.

179

Features	Analysis
On the day she had the current pain, she was at a medical symposium sponsored by her company. She had spent much of the last week preparing material for the meeting but had been well. An hour before the pain started, she had had a heavy lunch and drunk a lot of mineral water. The pain started gradually and was located in her right loin. Gradually, it built up to a peak within an hour and was constant and severe. 'It was possibly the worst pain I have ever had'. The pain radiated to her back, on the right, 'a few inches below the shoulder blade'. It also radiated down to her right iliac fossa and suprapubic area but not to her perineum or thigh.	Loin pain starting within an hour of a high fluid intake is typical of renal tract obstruction. The renal pelvis distends when the kidney excretes urine rapidly and causes pain. She had also had a heavy meal, and this should make us think of gall bladder disease. The location and radiation of this pain make either disease possible, but on balance, renal tract disease is more likely. Note that this lady's pain is not 'colic'.
	Most authorities do not believe that pain from renal or biliary obstruction is true colic, and the symptoms described by this lady are more typical of renal or biliary obstruction.
The pain made her roll around in agony but she could not find a comfortable position. There were no apparent aggravating factors. The pain started to improve an hour after she was given an intramuscular injection of 100 mg pethidine but did not subside completely till 6 hours later.	Gynaecological disease (e.g. torsion of an ovarian cyst and rupture of ectopic pregnancy) and appendicitis, though much less likely, cannot be ruled out absolutely at this stage.
She had nausea and vomited most of the food she had eaten during lunch. There was no blood in the vomit. She felt a bit hot and shivery when the pain was severe.	Nausea and vomiting do not have a high diagnostic value as they occur commonly in a wide variety of acute acute abdominal disorders.

Detailed systems review did not reveal other symptoms. In particular, she denied frequency of micturition, pain or difficulty passing urine and haematuria. Her bowels and periods were regular. Her last menstrual period was 3 weeks before and she had no vaginal discharge. She had an intrauterine contraceptive device (IUCD) in place and it was fitted a year before. She never had pain with her periods.

Absence of urinary or gynaecological symptoms does not of course exclude disease in these systems.

She had no significant illnesses in the past and was not taking regular medications. There was no history of kidney or other disorders in her family.

There are no further clues for making a firm diagnosis on the past medical, drug and family history.

On examination she looked well but was obviously in pain and distress. She was afebrile and was not anaemic or jaundiced, and was well hydrated.

If the renal tract is obstructed, there is a risk of infection. Fever, rigors and a raised temperature suggest infection. They are absent but the urine must be cultured.

BP was 120/70, pulse 96/min and regular. Examination of the head, neck and chest showed no abnormalities. The breasts and axillae were normal.

Abdominal examination showed no scars, distension or masses. She was tender and had guarding in the right loin, renal angle and right upper quadrant. The liver, kidneys and spleen were not palpable. Bowel sounds were normal and there were no bruits. Hernial orifices were intact and there were no groin lymph nodes. Vaginal and rectal examinations were normal.

Abdominal and pelvic examination allows us to narrow the diagnostic probabilities. Renal tract disease is now more probable from the site of tenderness and guarding, but again, do not discount appendicitis and gall bladder disease or ectopic pregnancy.

181

Features	*Analysis*

Clinical diagnosis

The most likely diagnosis is stone in the renal pelvis or ureter as yet probably not complicated by infection. In favour of this are the past history of similar though milder pain and the characteristics of the acute pain (discussed above). Less probable are acute appendicitis and acute cholecystitis.

Investigations

Urinalysis showed a moderate amount of red cells; there was no bilirubin or urobilinogen. Urine culture was negative.	This suggests a disease process in the urinary tract, for instance ureteric stone, or one next to the urinary tract, e.g. an inflamed appendix lying next to the urinary bladder. It is important for the urine to be collected and tested properly.
Pregnancy test was negative.	Pregnancy test may be negative in early pregnancy.
Hb, U&Es and LFTs were normal Plain X-ray of her abdomen, including the kidney and urinary bladder (KUB), did not reveal any abnormalities.	These negative blood tests and X-ray do not rule out renal or gall stones, as stated earlier. She has an IUCD in place and a negative pregnancy test, making pregnancy unlikely. As a rule, however, you must be satisfied that a young woman is not pregnant before taking X-rays of her abdomen and pelvis. If you suspect gall stones, tell the radiographer so that he can take special views of the gall bladder area.

IVU showed delayed excretion from the right kidney and dilatation of the renal pelvis and ureter to just above the uretero-vesical junction. The features were those of a calculus obstructing the right ureter.

Final diagnosis
Right ureteric calculus.

It is important to exclude a cause for her ureteric calculus such as hyperparathyroidism. Any stones passed should be analysed.

Chapter 12

Haematuria

Haematuria is the passage of urine containing three or more red blood cells per high power field. The patient may complain of passing blood in his urine if the quantity of blood is large enough to be seen with the naked eye. Haematuria demands full urological investigation as it may be due to carcinoma in the bladder. If, however, microscopic haematuria is discovered on routine urinalysis, there is no general agreement about the extent of investigation necessary.

Before extensive investigations are embarked upon, it is useful to determine by microscopy whether the red colour of the urine is due to blood. Beetroot and phenolphthalein-containing laxatives colour the urine red.

Causes of haematuria (commoner causes indicated by *)

These can be (a) general and (b) local.

(a) General causes of haematuria:
    These include haemorrhagic disorders and anti-coagulant medication.*

(b) Local causes of haematuria:
    (i) In the kidney – neoplasm*
                           – stone*
                           – injury*
                           – infection such as pyelonephritis or pyonephrosis*
                           – glomerulonephritis
                           – polycystic disease
                           – TB
    (ii) In the ureter – neoplasm
                           – stone*
    (iii) In the bladder – neoplasm*
                           – infection*
                           – stone
                           – foreign body
                           – injury*
    (iv) In the prostate – benign hyperplasia*
                           – neoplasm*
                           – infection*

(v) In the urethra – injury
                     – infection*
                     – neoplasm

Commonest causes

Infections (50%), urinary tract calculi (15%), injuries (10%), prostatic hyperplasia (10%), neoplasms of the urinary tract (5%).

Points to look for

You will note that many of the causes of haematuria are similar to those of urinary tract pain; they will not be dealt with again.

Malignancy of the urinary tract

The main reason for investigating haematuria thoroughly is to be sure that malignancy is not missed. The main symptoms of renal carcinoma are haematuria, renal angle pain and lethargy due to anaemia. Signs include a renal mass and hypertension but may be absent. By contrast, bladder carcinoma presents in most cases with painless haematuria. In a patient who bleeds severely, acute retention of urine may occur from obstruction of the urethra by clot, but this is not a common presentation of bladder tumour. Other presentations include hydronephrosis due to obstruction of one ureter or (rarely) uraemia from obstruction of both ureters.

Prostatic disease

This is a common cause of haematuria in men. Benign hyperplasia causes bleeding more often than malignancy of the prostate. Symptoms of bladder outflow obstruction are common. Malignancy can sometimes be diagnosed on rectal examination.

History

Reason for question	Question asked	Comment
Find out if there has been haematuria in the past	Have you ever passed blood in your water before now? If yes find out all about the investigations done (if any), the results and the action that was taken	
Find out more about this episode	When did you first notice that there was something wrong with your water (or urine)?	
	What did you notice wrong?	The patient will tell you that he noticed blood in his urine but at least give him a chance to volunteer this information
Urinary tract or vaginal bleeding?	In a woman, was the blood in the urine or was it from the front passage or the vagina?	Make sure it is haematuria not vaginal bleeding
	Have you noticed blood in your water every time you have passed water?	Most haematuria is episodic rather than continuous
How much blood?	How heavily blood-stained is the urine? Describe the colour of the urine (for instance like rosé or claret). Are there any clots in it?	If the amount of blood is large the urine is red and thick and sometimes has clots in it

Source of the blood	When in the course of the urine stream do you notice the blood? Throughout the stream, (total haematuria), at the beginning (initial haematuria) or at the end (terminal haematuria)? Do you see blood on your underclothes?	In general, total haematuria is due to bleeding from the upper tract (kidney or ureter); initial haematuria suggests an origin from the bladder neck, prostate or urethra. Terminal haematuria suggests a lesion in the bladder. Blood from the distal part of the urethra can stain the underclothes, but be sure it is not from the rectum or vagina
Associated symptoms may give a clue to the cause of the bleeding	Do you get any pain with the bleeding?	Haematuria without pain is more ominous than when associated with pain and should raise suspicion about a neoplasm in the kidney or bladder
	If yes, find out the nature of the pain and decide whether it is fixed renal pain, renal colic or strangury (see previous chapter)	Haematuria with fixed renal pain or renal colic suggests a stone in the kidney or ureter; with strangury it suggests a bladder stone or passage of blood clots
	How often do you have the urge to pass urine? Is this more often than usual? Does the water sting or burn when you pass it?	Haematuria with frequency and burning on micturition may be due to infection
	Symptoms of bladder outflow obstruction (see Chapter 13)	These suggest the cause is an enlarged prostate in a man but does not exclude bladder carcinoma
	Do you bruise easily or bleed unduly when you cut yourself?	Think of a clotting disorder as the cause of the bleeding

Reason for question	Question asked	Comment
ROS	RS: Cough, sputum, haemoptysis, dyspnoea, pleuritic chest pain?	Any suggestion of secondaries in the lungs?
	CVS, GIT	Uraemia can cause anorexia, tiredness and weight loss
	CNS	Uraemia or secondaries in the brain may give rise to CNS symptoms such as fits, headaches and drowsiness
PMH	Previous urinary tract disease such as stones, infection, neoplasm?	
	History of injury?	
DRUGS	Anticoagulants	These increase the likelihood of bleeding
	Phenolphthalein-containing laxatives	These can colour urine red
	Non-steroidal anti-inflammatory drugs	These can cause haematuria. One NSAID in particular, tiaprofenic acid (Surgam), has been reported to cause haematuria (and other urinary symptoms) more often than others
	Cytotoxic chemotherapy	
SH	Smoking	Causes urinary tract malignancies
	Occupation	A full occupational history is mandatory in a patient with bladder cancer. The patient is entitled to compensation if bladder cancer was caused by working with chemicals such as aniline dyes, or in the rubber industries

188

| *FH* | Family history of renal disease, especially polycystic disease; family history of bleeding disorders, or urinary tract calculi | |

ALLERGIES

Examination

General examination	As for 'Urinary tract pain' (previous chapter) including: bruises (ask if they came on spontaneously or after injury)	Anticoagulant therapy or clotting disorder
RS *CVS* *CNS* *ABDOMEN*	As for 'Urinary tract pain' in previous chapter Abdominal examination includes rectal and pelvic examination as for renal tract pain	The important point here is to make sure that malignancy is not missed

Investigations

The investigation of the patient with haematuria is identical in many respects to that of the patient with renal tract pain as outlined above. To help rule out prostate malignancy, serum prostate specific antigen (PSA) should be measured. The important difference is that haematuria is more often due to malignancy than is urinary tract pain. All patients with haematuria should be investigated up to 'IVU' as in the last chapter and should also have cystoscopy. If a bladder neoplasm is found, it should be resected completely if possible and sent for histology. A malignant prostate will require biopsy, or resection if the patient has bladder outflow symptoms. This will not only provide histological material, but it will relieve outflow obstruction. Some workers claim that resection of prostate cancer adversely affects survival.

Case report

Features	Analysis
Mr Frank Drummer is aged 69. He is a retired car mechanic and lives with his wife and one unmarried son. He was referred urgently by his GP because of a 2-week history of painless haematuria.	Haematuria always demands urgent and full investigation. At this age there is a high risk of malignancy of the urinary tract.
He had retired at the age of 60 because of arthritis of both knees and was taking NSAIDs, but was otherwise well. He had never passed blood in his urine before. One morning 2 weeks before he saw his GP, he passed blood in his urine for no apparent reason. The urine was heavily blood stained but more so towards the end of micturition. He described the colour of the blood as bright red. He had had no pain while passing urine.	As pointed out above, NSAIDs can cause haematuria, but often with other lower urinary symptoms such as frequency and pain, due to bladder irritation. Haematuria more profuse towards the end of micturition suggests a lesion in the bladder such as tumour, but do not rely on the localizing value of this finding. Painless haematuria is highly suggestive of malignancy.

He had passed blood on three further occasions since. For the last 3 years, he has had the urge to pass urine more often than before and when he has to go he has to rush. The urine does not come immediately and he has to wait a few seconds longer and uses slightly more force to empty his bladder than before. He dribbles slightly at the end.

The symptoms indicate bladder outflow obstruction but this must be confirmed by tests (see Chapter 13). The likely cause is prostatic enlargement, but, even if this is present, bleeding must not be ascribed to it until the whole urinary tract has been fully investigated.

He did not bruise easily or bleed unduly following minor trauma. He had had an early morning cough for the last 6 months and expectorated yellow mucoid sputum, perhaps half a teaspoonful each morning.

This is the so-called 'smoker's cough' but note that there is a higher risk of cancers of the lung and bladder in smokers compared with non-smokers.

He walked with the aid of a walking stick as he had arthritis of both knees, but was able to get about. He had no other symptoms on systems review.

Systems review is important so as not to miss symptoms due to metastatic disease. It may also uncover other possible causes of bleeding.

He took Brufen tablets, 200 mg three times daily for his arthritis and had good control of his pain from them. He was on no other medications.

NSAIDs, as mentioned above, can cause bladder irritation and haematuria.

He smoked 20 cigarettes a day from the age of 18 and drank 12 units of alcohol a week. He worked as a shop assistant and then as a motor mechanic most of his life and had never worked in the chemical industry or handled dangerous chemicals. There was no family history of kidney or other diseases.

The increased risk of bladder cancer in smokers has been mentioned above. A full occupational history is important if bladder cancer is suspected or confirmed.

Features	*Analysis*
He looked well but was obviously overweight; his weight was 87 kg and his height 1.67 metres (5 ft 6 in). He was not anaemic, cyanosed or jaundiced and had no finger clubbing. His fingers were nicotine stained.	Symptoms from arthritis of the knees are made worse by obesity. He should be advised to lose weight. Nicotine staining of his fingers corroborates the long history of smoking.
There were no abnormalities in his head or neck, in particular no enlarged lymph nodes. His chest was clear and his heart normal on clinical examination. BP was 150/95 and pulse 88/min and regular. Peripheral pulses were all present and normal.	Physical examination often does not reveal any abnormalities in bladder carcinoma.
Examination of the abdomen and groins was normal. Specifically, the liver was not enlarged and there were no masses. Kidneys and bladder were not palpable and his genitalia were normal. Rectal examination showed a moderately enlarged prostate, which felt benign. There were no other abnormalities. Neurological examination did not reveal any abnormalities.	You must examine for abnormalities of urinary organs, from kidneys to bladder. The only clinical abnormality is an enlarged prostate, but bladder cancer may also be present.
Examination of his locomotor system showed reduction in movement of both knees and crepitus in the right. Other joints were normal.	In keeping with osteoarthritis of the knees.

Clinical diagnosis

Benign prostatic hyperplasia causes haematuria but bladder carcinoma is also highly likely. In a patient of this age, the rule of thumb is that bladder cancer *IS* the diagnosis unless proved otherwise by full urological investigation including cystoscopy.

Investigations
Urinalysis showed a large amount of red cells but culture was negative.
Hb was 13.5 g/dl, WCC, ESR, U&Es, LFTs normal.
Urine cytology showed malignant cells.
Chest X-ray was normal. Ultrasound of the abdomen showed normal kidneys, liver, biliary tract and pancreas.

IVU showed a filling defect on the right side of the bladder.
Cystoscopy revealed a polypoid mass at the site of the filling defect in the bladder. The ureteric orifice was not involved. Most of the visible tumour was resected but bimanual examination of the bladder under general anaesthetic showed a nodule at the site.

Urine cytology is a useful test and can be carried out while waiting to do cystoscopy. Cells from a tumour in the urinary tract are shed intermittently in the urine and can be seen on cytology. Biopsy is needed to determine the nature of the tumour.

The presence of a thickening after excision of visible tumour suggests bladder muscle invasion by tumour. In this examination, the surgeon puts the index finger of one hand in the patient's rectum and then presses on the bladder with the fingers of the other hand placed firmly on the suprapubic region. The thickening, if present, is felt between the two hands.

Biopsy showed a transitional cell carcinoma of the bladder.

Final diagnosis
Transitional cell carcinoma of the bladder, invading the bladder muscle.

Chapter 13

Acute urinary retention in a man

Acute retention of urine is a surgical emergency for three reasons:

(a) It is a painful condition. This is in contrast to chronic retention, which is painless and is often discovered incidentally.
(b) It can lead to urinary tract infection.
(c) It can cause uraemia, especially if there is long standing obstruction.

Causes of acute retention of urine

Acute retention is most commonly due to disease or obstruction of (a) the prostate. (b) The urethra is a rare cause and is mentioned for completeness. Retention can also result from (c) acute neurological damage such as transection of the cord and (d) after injury or an operation in the groin or perineum. There is a high risk of urethral damage in pelvic fracture. (e) Drugs which affect the autonomic nervous system can also cause retention of urine. In elderly patients (f) constipation is a common precipitating event.

Although the comments here apply mainly to retention due to (a) and (b), the others must be remembered.

(a) The prostate
   (i) Benign hyperplasia.
   (ii) Carcinoma of the prostate.
(b) The urethra
   (i) Causes in the lumen: calculi, foreign bodies, blood clot e.g. following injury.
   (ii) Causes in the wall: e.g. following instrumentation and venereal disease. This cause of retention is rare.
   (iii) Outside the wall: periurethral abscess or haematoma.

Common causes of acute retention of urine

Benign hyperplasia of prostate (70%), carcinoma of

prostate (10%), following operations on the groin or perineum (10%), urethral stricture (2%).

Points to look for

Men who present with symptoms suggesting progressive obstruction of urinary flow are often said to have 'prostatic symptoms' or 'prostatism'. While disease of the prostate is the commonest cause of such symptoms it is by no means the only one. Such symptoms are also very common in elderly women. It has been suggested that these symptoms are better referred to as 'bladder outflow symptoms' or 'obstructive urinary symptoms', but even these terms are not precise. Only two-thirds of patients with these symptoms have objective evidence of obstruction.

The other type of lower urinary disturbance is characterized by what are referred to as 'irritative' symptoms. Irritative implies a pathological process such as infection, stone or tumour but this is not the case. Irritative symptoms almost always indicate an abnormality of detrusor (bladder muscle) function.

Obstructive and irritative symptoms are frequently present in a patient with prostatic enlargement, but irritative symptoms may be present without bladder outflow obstruction. A patient with irritative symptoms will not benefit from prostatectomy.

In an editorial in the *British Medical Journal*, Abrams (1994) suggests 'voiding' and 'filling' symptoms to replace 'obstructive' and 'irritative' respectively, as these terms describe a patient's symptoms without implying their cause. I suggest you read this paper.

Despite the above misgivings, I have retained the terms 'obstructive' and 'irritative' as they are more widely used at the moment. However, the student must recognize their limitations and every patient with lower urinary symptoms must have objective investigations such as urine flow rate measurement.

Obstructive and irritative symptoms

Obstructive symptoms are:
 –difficulty initiating micturition (hesitancy)
 –poor stream; the patient may have to strain hard to empty his bladder and may take several minutes to complete micturition
 –dribbling at the end of micturition

It may be possible to distinguish obstructive from irritative bladder symptoms. The latter include:

- frequency of micturition
- nocturia
- sudden desire to pass urine, which if not heeded, results in incontinence (urgency)

Obstructive symptoms due to an enlarged prostate are present for many months or even years before acute retention. Some patients present non-urgently for investigation of these symptoms, while others may be seen for the first time after they develop acute retention. Some patients develop acute retention following operations.

The scheme described here can be modified for the investigation of the patient who presents to the outpatient clinic with bladder outflow symptoms but is not in urinary retention.

Initial management

The first treatment of a patient who presents with acute retention of urine is bladder catheterization. This should not be delayed while the history is obtained or blood tests done. A history of inability to pass urine with pain is enough. Examination involves inspecting, palpating and percussing gently the abdomen to discover if the bladder is distended. Beware the patient with a large painful abdominal aortic aneurysm who has become anuric.

NOTE THE EASE WITH WHICH THE CATHETER CAN BE PASSED (difficult catheterization may be due to the operator being inexperienced but could be due to stricture of the urethra, stone in the urethra or enlarged prostate). In the event of more than mild difficulty of catheterization consideration should be given to the percutaneous insertion of a suprapubic catheter.

History

Reason for question	Question asked	Comment
Establish duration of retention	When did you last pass urine?	

Events leading up to retention, possible cause of acute event	How did the stoppage happen? Had you been out for a drink, or out in cold weather? Have you been taking any new medicines?	All the factors here can interfere with detrusor function. Enquire about drugs that interfere with autonomic nerve function, e.g. antidepressants
	Had you had an injury or an operation in your groin or around your back passage area?	Common operations that result in acute retention of urine are groin hernia repair, haemorrhoidectomy, drainage of perianal abscess
	How have your bowels been? Has there been any change in your bowel habit?	Constipation is a common cause of acute retention of urine but not on its own. Impacted faeces may precipitate retention when the patient already has prostatic obstruction
Distinguish between symptoms of bladder 'irritation' and bladder of outflow obstruction	*Irritative symptoms:* How often do you get the urge to pass urine in the day? How many times do you get up in the night to pass urine?	Note diurnal frequency of micturition as number of hours from one voiding to the next and nocturnal frequency as number of times the patient voids at night e.g. 2 hourly/4
	When you have to go to pass urine, do you have to rush? If you did not go, what would happen? Would you wet yourself?	Document whether urgency of micturition present

197

Reason for question	Question asked	Comment
	Obstructive symptoms:	
	When you get there, does the water come straight away or do you have to wait some time? How long?	Hesitancy, measured in seconds, is an important symptom of outflow obstruction. In general, the longer the time, the greater the degree of obstruction
	When the water comes, what is the flow like, compared to say 10 years ago?	Reduction in the force of the stream is one of the most reliable symptoms of outflow obstruction
	How hard do you have to strain to pass urine? How much force do you have to apply to pass urine? Do you get short of breath trying to pass urine?	Increasing force to pass urine, grunting and shortness of breath while passing urine are all indicative of severe outflow obstruction
	What happens when you think you have finished passing water? Do you dribble? Do you feel as though you could go again straight away?	Dribbling indicates obstruction
Associated symptoms	Any pain? If yes find out all you can about it	Pain in the perineum, over the sacrum, or in the rectum, may be due to prostatitis or prostatic carcinoma
		Stinging or burning pain on micturition may be due to urinary tract infection or to urethritis
		Bone pain should alert you to secondary deposits from carcinoma, especially of the prostate

	Have you passed any blood in your water?	While haematuria may be due to benign hyperplasia of the prostate, its presence demands full investigation to exclude carcinoma in the urinary tract
ROS	Rest of GUS, RS, CVS, GIT	
	CNS	Neurological disease can cause acute and chronic retention of urine
PMH	Instrumentation, e.g. cystoscopy, catheterization Other urological operations such as prostatectomy Urethral infection, e.g. venereal disease Injury involving the pelvis	These can cause injury to the urethra which heals by fibrosis and thus develops a stricture
	Recent circumcision	Meatal stenosis can result from this operation
	Recent groin or perineal operations (see above)	Retention of urine more likely in a patient with previous obstructive symptoms
FH, SH		
DRUGS	Cold/cough medications; antidepressants; anaesthetic agents	Can cause acute retention of urine
ALLERGIES		

Examination

Reason for examination	*Sign elicited*	*Comment*
General condition	The patient with uncomplicated acute retention of urine is often elderly, and may well have other medical problems. He may have developed retention when put to bed for some other problem, for instance heart failure, or following an operation. He will be in pain and distress from the distended bladder. Pain will dictate the urgency with which the patient should be catheterized. He will stop drinking for fear of distending the bladder more and so you must assess his state of hydration. If the patient is anaemic, think of carcinoma of the prostate or uraemia.	
Any signs of uraemia?	There is a high chance of uraemia in a patient who is drowsy or confused, restless or twitching.	
RS	Signs of lung collapse, consolidation or pleural effusion	Suggesting secondary deposits in lungs from urinary tract malignancy
CVS		
CNS		CNS signs may be due to secondary carcinoma or uraemia. CNS lesions can cause urinary retention as indicated above. Uraemia may cause fits

Scars from previous urinary and other operations.	Especially prostatectomy
Is the abdomen distended?	Bladder should no longer be distended if the catheter is draining well
Tenderness (especially in renal angle)	May be from renal tract infection
Abdominal masses	Possibility of tumour deposits
Liver enlarged	Hepatomegaly due to secondary deposits
Kidneys enlarged	Think of hydronephrosis from bladder outflow obstruction
Examine genitalia. Any urethral discharge?	Suggests venereal infection
Look at penile meatus, or if foreskin present, at foreskin meatus as well, especially if urethral catheterization was difficult	Either meatus could be stenosed
Oedema of the legs	Lymphoedema may be due to obstruction of lymphatics by malignant lymph nodes; pitting oedema due to obstruction of major veins
PR: bladder should be empty. Any tenderness?	Think of prostatitis or anal abscess
Any masses/nodules?	For instance, carcinoma of prostate but only if disease is locally widespread

Reason for examination	Sign elicited	Comment
	Examine the prostate carefully	You will often see in case notes statements such as 'Prostate moderately enlarged ...' It is important to realize that prostatic size cannot be judged accurately by rectal examination in the conscious patient. Moreover, prostatic size does not correlate with severity of outflow symptoms
	Does the gland feel firm and rubbery, and can the median sulcus be palpated? Can the rectal mucosa be moved over the gland?	These are the features of benign hyperplasia
	Or is the gland hard and irregular? Is the rectal mucosa infiltrated?	These are features of advanced carcinoma of the prostate
	Are there any other masses within or outside the rectum?	Spread of prostatic carcinoma
	Any blood on the glove finger stall?	Ulcerated carcinoma of the rectum
MUSCULO-SKELETAL	Any bone tenderness or diminished joint movement?	This suggests bony metastases from prostatic cancer

Investigations

Patients who do not require investigation

Not every patient with acute retention of urine requires investigation: for example, a patient without previous obstructive urinary symptoms, who, after a groin or perianal operation, develops retention. Usually he will pass urine when pain from the operation subsides and the catheter is removed.

Those who require investigation

In the remaining patients, tests are carried out for two reasons:

(a) To determine the cause of the acute retention.
(b) To determine whether any complications have occurred from urinary obstruction. The most important are (i) uraemia and (ii) infection of the urinary tract.

These patients should all have urine microscopy, culture and sensitivity, blood count, urea, electrolytes and creatinine.

Further tests depend on the condition suspected.

Benign prostatic hyperplasia

Ultrasound of the urinary tract.
Other investigations: urodynamics if a neurological cause is suspected.

Carcinoma of the prostate

Prostatic carcinoma is often diagnosed incidentally. One common way in which it is diagnosed is from histology in a patient who has undergone prostatectomy for presumed benign hyperplasia.

If the condition is suspected from the clinical findings (e.g. a hard, irregular prostate), one way to confirm the diagnosis is to take a biopsy using a large bore needle (Tru-cut) introduced through the perineum or the rectum and to examine the specimen obtained histologically.

Transrectal ultrasound has helped to make this more accurate.

Other investigations: serum prostatic specific antigen, X-rays of the pelvis and chest, isotope bone scan.

Urethrogram, flexible cystoscopy.

Interpretation of tests in acute retention of urine

Urine examination: Look at the urine. Does it look cloudy or blood stained? Is there gravel or other sediment? Blood in the urine may be due to the trauma of catheterization.

Urine microscopy and culture: Note the number of white cells per field; if there are no white cells in the urine, bacteria present are due to contamination and not to infection. If organisms are cultured they will be identified and where indicated their bacterial sensitivities will be determined.

Hb: Anaemia may be present in malignancies of the urinary tract or in chronic renal failure.

WCC: This may be raised when infection is present.

ESR: This may be raised if there is tumour or bacterial infection.

Urea, electrolytes and creatinine: These are useful tests of renal function. Raised urea and creatinine may be due to reduced renal function as a result of long-standing obstruction.

Serum prostatic specific antigen: This is present in blood in some patients with carcinoma of the prostate and levels are raised in those with metastatic disease. It does not rise following rectal examination. Normal levels are found in prostatic carcinoma and it is therefore not a useful screening test.

X-ray of the chest: The chest X-ray may show secondary tumour or chest infection.

IVU: The role of IVU in the investigation of the patient presenting with bladder outflow symptoms and acute retention of urine has changed over the last few years, in that it is performed far less frequently. All the information that is given by the IVU can be obtained from ultrasound, which is safer and does not involve radiation and injection of contrast.

Ultrasound: This is an important and non-invasive method of investigating the urinary tract from the kidneys to the prostate. It can show the following:

Kidneys: mass lesions such as tumours, cysts,
dilatation of the pelvis and calyces from obstruction
absence of a kidney, for example due to agenesis or following surgical removal
the thickness of the renal cortex; the cortex gets thinner when the kidney is chronically obstructed.
the kidneys are small in chronic renal failure

Ureters: dilatation in obstruction

Bladder: tumours; volume of the bladder

Prostate: size and presence of tumour

Urinary flow rates: This is an important test in those with suspected outflow obstruction *but not in acute retention.* It measures the rate at which the patient empties a full bladder, and the values obtained correlate well with the degree of obstruction. It is useful in distinguishing between those patients with irritative symptoms from those with outflow obstruction.

Flow rate is measured electronically. The patient first drinks 2 litres of water and waits until his bladder is full. He then voids into a container placed on top of a measuring device connected to a transducer. The weight of urine is converted to volume and recorded on a chart in ml per second (Fig 13.1a). A normal pattern is represented by a bell-shaped curve (Fig 13.1b). Abnormal flow patterns are shown. In a patient with bladder outlet obstruction, maximum and average flow rates are diminished and flow time prolonged (Fig 13.1c). The voided volume (the area under the curve) is reduced. Other flow problems such as a hypocontractile detrusor, are difficult to diagnose in flow studies and require urodynamics.

Cystoscopy: This is done routinely in patients having endoscopic procedures for acute retention. It will detect or confirm strictures of the urethra, the extent of enlargement of the prostate into the urethra and the bladder, and the presence of bladder carcinoma. The bladder is emptied and the size of the prostate assessed by bimanual examination.

Urodynamics: Diseases such as an unstable bladder and neurological lesions affecting the nerve supply to the bladder may produce symptoms suggesting bladder outflow obstruction. It is important to identify or exclude these diseases because their management is different. Urodynamics is a means of

Urinary Flow Rate (UFR)

- UFR is the product of detrusor action against outlet resistance.
- The normal flow rate from a full bladder is about 20–25 ml/s in men and 25–30 ml/s in women.
- The variations are directly related to the volume voided and the subject's age.
- Obstruction should be suspected in any adult voiding with a full bladder at a rate of less than 15 ml/s. A flow rate of < 10 ml/s is considered definite evidence of obstruction.

Procedure

The flow rate is recorded electronically. The patient, after drinking 3 pints of water and achieving a full bladder, voids into a container on top of a measuring device that is connected to a transducer, the weight being converted to volume and recorded on a chart in ml/s.

Interpretation

- Evaluation should include at least two flow events.
- In an adult, flow volume of < 150 ml should be interpreted with caution.
- A *normal pattern* is represented by a bell-shaped curve.

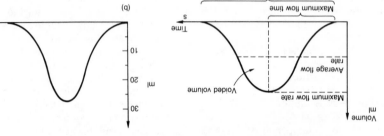

(a)

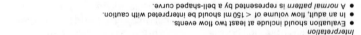

(b)

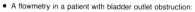

- A flowmetry in a patient with bladder outlet obstruction:

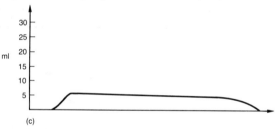

(c)

Figure 13.1. *Urine flow rate measurement. The weight of urine is converted to volume (a). The normal pattern (b) is represented by a bell-shaped curve. In bladder outlet obstruction (c) the maximum and average flow rates are reduced and flow time prolonged*

investigating the function of the bladder, the bladder neck and urethra by measuring bladder pressures during filling and emptying; it also measures urine flow rates.

The patient empties his bladder and a two-way catheter is inserted. Any residual urine is measured. One limb of the catheter is attached to a reservoir of fluid and the other to a pressure recorder. The pressures recorded from the bladder represent the activity of the detrusor muscle and the pressure exerted from the abdomen. The latter is measured with a probe inserted in the rectum and subtracted from the bladder pressure readings. Warm fluid is run into the bladder until the patient feels a desire to micturate. The volume required is termed the filling volume and is normally 400 ml, but may be more. Pressures are recorded as the patient voids. Flow rate can also be measured, and it gives an indication of bladder muscle contractility and urethral resistance.

Urethrogram: Urethral stricture is confirmed by failed catheterization, and a urethrogram is usually only done in those with complex urethral strictures. Contrast medium is injected into the urethra through a catheter introduced through the penile meatus. X-rays are taken of the urethra and the bladder.

Case report

Features	Analysis
Mr Mohammed Said is aged 78 and is a retired diplomat. He lives with his married daughter and her family. He presented to the accident and emergency department because he could not pass urine for 24 hours.	Prostatic obstruction is the commonest cause of acute retention of urine in a man of 78 but do not ignore other possible causes. A catheter must be inserted at the earliest opportunity, once it is confirmed that the patient has acute retention of urine, and the amount of urine drained immediately through the catheter should be recorded. The rest of the history and examination can wait.

He admitted that his water works had not been right for over 10 years, but had learned to live with his symptoms. During this time, he had had progressive irritative and obstructive bladder symptoms. The former were frequency of micturition and a sudden desire to pass urine. He passed urine every 3 hours in the day and woke up 3 times at night to empty his bladder. When he had the urge to pass urine and did not go immediately, he often wet himself. Obstructive symptoms were equally troublesome. He had had difficulty initiating micturition and usually waited about 15 seconds before he could start passing urine. When urine started to flow, he had to exert a lot of force to maintain the stream, and dribbled at the end.

Irritative and obstructive bladder symptoms are present in up to 80% of elderly men and in more than 95% of those presenting spontaneously with acute retention of urine. The significance of these symptoms is discussed above; they tell us little about the underlying cause.

The day before he presented to hospital, he had been out with his daughter and son-in-law to a restaurant to celebrate his 78th birthday. He remembered emptying his bladder before he left and drank a fair amount of mineral water during the meal. When he arrived home, he tried to pass urine before he went to bed but could not. He was also surprised that he had gone through the night without getting up to pass urine. He kept trying unsuccessfully the whole day to pass urine. Late in the evening, he developed severe pain in the suprapubic region and asked his daughter to take him to hospital.

In many patients with progressive bladder outflow obstruction, there is a precipitating cause for acute retention. Examples are a higher than usual fluid intake, an operation, constipation, an episode of confusion, specific drug therapy and an acute illness.

Features	Analysis
He denied haematuria, pain on micturition or urethral discharge.	Prostatic enlargement can cause haematuria, but, if this symptom is present, it should not be ascribed to the prostate until other more serious causes such as bladder carcinoma have been excluded.
Systems review revealed nothing remarkable. His bowels were regular.	An important cause of prostatic enlargement is carcinoma. Complications of urinary obstruction are urinary tract infection and uraemia. An attempt must be made to uncover these disorders in systems review.
He had not been on regular medication. He had malaria when he was a diplomat in East Africa years before but had had no other serious illnesses or operations. He had never had urethral operations or catheterization.	As mentioned above, drugs and operation can cause urinary obstruction.
On examination, he was in great distress but looked well for his age. He was well orientated in person, time and place. He was not anaemic or jaundiced and was well hydrated. His temperature was normal.	Be aware of uraemia and urinary infection as complications of urinary retention.
BP was 170/115 and pulse 96/min and regular. Peripheral pulses were all present and normal. Clinical examination of the heart and lungs showed no abnormalities. The abdomen was soft. The bladder was distended almost up to his umbilicus and was tender on palpation. There were no other masses and liver, kidneys and spleen were not palpable. Rectal examination was deferred until after catheterization.	The BP is raised but this may be due to the patient's distress. Check it again when he has been catheterized and is free of pain.

Neurological examination was normal.

Rectal examination was carried out after the catheter was inserted. Soft faeces were present in the rectum. The prostate was moderately enlarged and felt smooth, rubbery and non-tender. No other masses were felt and there was no blood on the glove finger stall.

It is difficult to assess the prostate adequately when the bladder is full. Prostatic size cannot be measured reliably in a conscious patient. Clinically the prostate feels benign, but malignancy cannot be ruled out.

Clinical diagnosis

The most likely diagnosis is benign prostatic hyperplasia leading to acute retention of urine. A number of these patients have carcinoma of the prostate, which may only come to light after histological examination of excised prostate. Another cause of this man's symptoms could be benign stricture of the urethra, but there is little in the history to support this diagnosis.

The patient was catheterized and 1.5 litres of urine drained. He felt much more comfortable.

Investigations

Urinalysis: there were numerous red cells in the urine but culture was negative.

The blood was probably due to the trauma of catheter insertion but cystoscopy is mandatory to exclude bladder carcinoma.

Hb, WCC, ESR, U&Es, LFTs, prostatic specific antigen were normal.

Trial without catheter was not believed to be justified in a man with such long-standing history. Prostatectomy was discussed with him. He agreed to this operation, and 3 weeks later, he underwent cystoscopy and transurethral prostatectomy. Histology of the prostatic tissue removed showed benign hyperplasia. There was no evidence of malignancy.

Final diagnosis
Benign prostatic hyperplasia causing progressive bladder outflow obstruction and ultimately acute retention of urine.

Reference

Abrams, P. (1994) New words for old: lower urinary tract symptoms for 'prostatism'. *British Medical Journal*, **308**, 929–930.

Chapter 14

Swelling of the groin or scrotum

Lumps in the groin may be associated with disease of the genital organs. Also, groin lumps such as hernia may affect the genitalia. The examination of these areas is therefore discussed together.

Causes of groin swellings

(a) Swellings arising from within the skin:
  (i) Sebaceous cyst
(b) Swellings arising from the subcutaneous tissues
  (i) Lipoma
(c) Swellings arising from the inguinal canal
  (i) Inguinal hernia
  (ii) Hydrocele of the cord (or of the canal of Nuck in the female)
  (iii) Lipoma of the cord

(iv) Malignancy of the cord, usually a rhabdomyosarcoma, but this is rare
(d) Just outside the inguinal canal
  (i) Undescended or retractile testis in the male
  (ii) Lymph node
  (iii) Malignancy of cord (see (c) above)
(e) Arising distal to the inguinal ligament
  (i) Femoral hernia
  (ii) Saphena varix
  (iii) Femoral artery aneurysm
  (iv) Lymph nodes
  (v) Psoas abscess
(f) Arising from within the scrotum
  (i) Cysts of the epididymis
  (ii) Varicocele
  (iii) Tumours of the testis
  (iv) Hydrocele
  (v) Epididymitis

Commonest causes

Hernias (60%), lymph nodes (15%), hydrocele (10%), cyst of epididymis (5%) epididymitis (2%), varicocele (2%).

Rare but important

Carcinoma of the testis, undescended testis in child or adult; or retractile testis in a child.

Points to look for

By the end of this examination you should be able to diagnose practically all scrotal and groin lumps. The important point is to perform a systematic examination every time. It is tempting to try to make a diagnosis by eliciting few signs. While this is possible with experience, it is not advised.

Inguinal hernia

This is a common groin swelling. The patient usually complains of an intermittent swelling in the groin: it is absent when he first wakes up in the morning, and appears as he strains, lifts, coughs or exercises. The lump may sometimes be difficult to reduce, and it will then become painful. There may be a history of bowel obstruction which resolves when the lump reduces. The swelling is above the medial part of the inguinal ligament and, if reducible, there will be a cough impulse over it. Although the student is required to attempt to control the hernia by reducing it and occluding the deep inguinal ring, this test can be inaccurate in distinguishing indirect from direct hernia.

Femoral hernia

This is common in elderly women. The patient may never have noticed the swelling and may present because of abdominal pain. The lump lies below the medial part of the inguinal ligament and may or may not be reducible. It is always important to look for hernias in patients presenting with acute abdominal pain.

Lymph nodes in the groin

These can be distinguished from other groin swellings

by their location below the inguinal ligament, often lateral to the site of femoral hernia, their firmness, and the absence of a cough impulse over them. If a lymph node is found, the external genitalia, perineum and the lower limbs should be carefully examined for a source of infection or tumour. Other lymph nodes should also be examined, as should the abdomen for evidence of neoplasm or enlargement of the spleen.

An enlarged node of the femoral canal (Cloquet's node) is difficult to distinguish from a femoral hernia.

Hydrocele

Fluid collects in the tunica vaginalis, making it diffi-cult to palpate the testis separately from the swelling. The scrotal swelling is painless and you can get above it. It transilluminates.

Undescended and retractile testes

These are seen more commonly in children. If there is no testis in the scrotum and one is found in the groin, an attempt should be made to bring it down into the scrotum. A retractile testis can be brought down, whereas an undescended testis may be, but immedi-ately retracts.

History

Reason for question	Question asked	Comment
Locate the lump	Please can you show me with one finger where the lump is	
Find out more about it (see Introduction) and possibly about its cause	How long have you been aware of this lump?	
	Is it getting bigger, smaller, or is it staying the same size?	

Reason for question	Question asked	Comment
	Is it there all the time, or does it come and go? What makes it appear or get bigger?	Inguinal swellings often appear in the upright position or when the patient strains, and disappear when he lies flat. Ectopic testis also changes position
	Is it painful or does it hurt when you press it?	Inflammatory swellings such as some lymph nodes and epididymitis are painful. Most of the other swellings are painless. An incarcerated or strangulated hernia is painful
	Do you experience any aching or pain in the groin?	Hernias can be painful
	Has the lump discharged?	Sebaceous cysts occasionally discharge. Discharge may be due to an abscess
	Do you get any pain in your back? If yes find out more about it	Psoas abscess may originate in the spine
	How do you feel in yourself? Has your weight changed? Do you get any fever, rigors or night sweats?	Systemic systems may occur with TB (causing psoas abscess), with lymphoma or with testicular malignancy
	Do you do heavy lifting or straining?	Relevant if hernia is suspected

ROS	*GIT Intermittent obstructive bowel symptoms (colicky abdominal pain, vomiting)?*	These suggest intermittent obstruction of hernia
	RS, CNS	If respiratory or CNS symptoms present, think of secondary malignancy, for instance from testicular tumour
	CVS	
	GUS	Urinary symptoms may be due to urinary infection, causing epididymitis
PMH		Past history of TB if psoas abscess is suspected
	History of chronic bronchitis	Coughing may aggravate hernia
	Previous hernia repair	Think of recurrent hernia
	Previous vasectomy	May cause mild distension of the epididymis
FH		
SH	Occupation	Important if hernia is suspected, not only for diagnosis, but also for advise on work after operation. There is no evidence that prolonged abstention from work reduces hernia recurrence rate
DRUGS		
ALLERGIES		

Examination

Reason for examination	Sign elicited	Comment
General examination	Ill/well, obese/slim	
	Enlarged lymph nodes in neck or axilla	In association with enlarged inguinal nodes should raise the possibility of lymphoma or TB
RS	Signs of chronic obstructive airways disease	Obstructive airways disease can be associated with hernia
CVS		
CNS		Neurological signs may be due to tumour
ABDOMEN	Scars	For example, previous hernia repair
	If the abdomen is distended, is there obstruction or ascites?	If the hernia is irreducible, it is almost certainly the cause of the obstruction
	Masses	For instance para-aortic lymph nodes from testicular tumour or lymphoma
	Enlarged liver	Think of secondary carcinoma
	Enlarged spleen	Think of lymphoma

(Examination should be carried out with the patient first standing and then lying down)

You may wish to combine examination of the groin and genitalia together under inspection and palpation

They are separated here for convenience

Draw an imaginary line between the anterior superior iliac spine and the pubic tubercle	This corresponds roughly with the inguinal ligament
Inspection: if a swelling can be seen, where is it in relation to the inguinal ligament?	This will help narrow down the diagnosis, for instance, if below the medial third of the inguinal ligament it may be a femoral hernia, lymph node, saphena varix or psoas abscess
Ask the patient to cough: is the lump more prominent?	If yes, think of hernia or saphena varix
If hernia suspected ask the patient to reduce it. Do not try to reduce it yourself	It is important not to hurt the patient
Palpation: palpate the anterior superior iliac spine and pubic tubercle: the inguinal ligament runs between. Ask patient to cough again and see where the swelling is in relation to the ligament	Inguinal hernia lies above the medial part of the ligament, femoral hernia below the medial part of the ligament
Is the lump tender?	Inflamed inguinal lymph node or irreducible hernia
Test for cough impulse or thrill over the swelling	Hernia or saphena varix. No cough impulse over a hydrocele of cord

219

Reason for examination	Sign elicited	Comment
	What is the consistency of the lump?	Lymph nodes are firm or rubbery, but may be hard and craggy. Saphena varix is soft. Hydrocele of the cord is cystic
	Does lump pulsate?	Aneurysm of the femoral or iliac artery
	Does the lump transilluminate?	Hydrocele of cord or of canal of Nuck
	If there is a reducible inguinal hernia, can you control it by occluding the deep inguinal ring?	This test is unreliable for distinguishing between direct and indirect inguinal hernias but is still taught
	In the male, examine the penis and remember to look under the foreskin	Infection or neoplasm from these areas drains to the inguinal nodes
	Examine the lower limbs: any lymphoedema or pitting oedema?	Obstruction of the veins or lymphatics by nodes or tumour would produce oedema
	Any varicose veins?	These should be expected if saphena varix is present
	If there are palpable lymph nodes, is there any tumour or infection of lower limb? Careful examination is necessary	Think especially of malignant melanoma
	Look in the interdigital webs especially for pigmented lesions	
	Examine the sole of the foot. Are there any ulcers?	

Inspection: Are there any swellings in the scrotal skin?

Sebaceous cysts are common at this site

Is the scrotal skin well formed?

In a patient with undescended testis, the scrotal sac may not be properly formed

Palpation: Is there a testis in the scrotum?

If not, the lump in the groin is probably an undescended testis. Confirm by palpating again and see if it can be brought towards the scrotum. If yes, continue the examination

Can you get above it?

If not, it is a hernia in an adult or an infantile hydrocele in a child

Confirm the latter by transillumination. If yes, continue the examination

Can you feel the testis separately from the lump?

If not, the swelling is probably a hydrocele or varicocele. Confirm the former by transillumination; for the latter, look for the 'bags of worms' sign more prominent on straining. Varicoceles are nearly always left sided

If yes, continue examination

Where is the swelling? In the epididymis?

Yes: epididymal cyst if it is cystic. Probably tuberculous epididymitis if solid, but this is very rare. However, it is not uncommon to see a thickened epididymis in a resolving acute epididymitis after antibiotic therapy

Reason for examination	Sign elicited	Comment
	In the testis?	Yes: probably tumour
	Involving both testis and epididymis?	Yes: neoplasm if hard or firm and non-tender. Epididymitis if tender. But beware, tumour can present as a painful and tender swelling

Investigations

For the majority of groin and scrotal swellings no laboratory investigations are required. If lymph nodes (of uncertain cause) or a testicular neoplasm are found, further investigations should be done. In the former the aim is to determine a cause for the enlarged lymph nodes, and, in the latter, to find out if spread has occurred. Ultrasound can often provide useful information.

Case report

Features	Analysis
John Malola is a 21-year-old student reading business administration at university. He was referred by his GP because of a swelling in the right groin of 12 months' duration.	Hernias and lymph nodes are the commonest swellings in the groin at this age.

He noticed the swelling 12 months ago when he was having a shower after a game of rugby. It disappeared when he lay flat and was only apparent when he stood up or strained. The swelling was largely painless but occasionally he noticed some discomfort over it.

A swelling appearing when the individual stands up and disappearing when lies flat is typical of a hernia, but may be due to a saphena varix.

Two weeks before he went to his GP, he was weight lifting in the gymnasium when the lump became painful and would not reduce easily. He stopped, lay down and was able gently to push the swelling back in. The groin was uncomfortable but the pain settled. He had no vomiting, abdominal pain or constipation.

This episode increases the possibility of hernia. The most likely explanation is that the hernia had become irreducible temporarily during strenuous exercise, but was pushed back once he stopped straining.

He had had no cough or difficulty passing urine and his bowels remained regular. Systems review revealed no symptoms.

There are no symptoms to aggravate a hernia.

He had had no previous illnesses or operations and was not on regular medication.

He looked well and was of muscular build. He was not anaemic or jaundiced, and had no abnormalities in the head and neck. BP was 120/75 and pulse 72/min and regular. Heart and lungs were normal.

There are no apparent abnormalities on examination.

223

Features	Analysis
Abdominal examination showed no scars or distension and no tenderness. Groin examination revealed a non-tender swelling with a cough impulse above the medial part of the inguinal ligament. It did not move down into the scrotum and was easily reducible. The lump could be controlled by placing a finger over the deep inguinal ring. The penis, scrotum and testes were normal.	This is a reducible inguinal hernia. It is probably indirect but the test to distinguish a direct from an indirect hernia is not reliable. The genitalia must be examined in all patients with groin swellings.
He had no varicose veins or evidence of saphena varix in his legs.	

Clinical diagnosis
The characteristics are those of a fully reducible, indirect right inguinal hernia. No specific investigations were necessary and this diagnosis was confirmed at operation.

Chapter 15

Intermittent claudication

Includes rest pain and ischaemic changes in the lower limb

This term is used to describe pain in one or both legs, generally in the muscles of the calf, occurring after walking a certain distance, and disappearing with rest. It is due to inadequate arterial blood flow to the muscle. Pain in the lower limb can occur from a variety of causes such as lesions affecting the cauda equina, the lumbar vertebrae, the pelvic cavity, and the sciatic nerve. It is therefore important to establish first that the patient is suffering from intermittent claudication by asking three questions:

1. Where is the pain when it comes on? Claudication is clearly in muscle, either of the calf, the thigh or the buttocks.
2. What brings the pain on? Claudication occurs after exercise, except in severe cases when the pain occurs at rest. The distance walked before claudication occurs is termed *the claudication distance*.

3. What eases the pain? Claudication (except, of course, ischaemic rest pain) is eased by rest.

History and examination enable the site of the arterial block to be predicted correctly in the majority of patients. Investigation helps to confirm the clinical diagnosis and is useful when an operation is contemplated. You must ensure first that it is claudication pain that limits the patient's exercise tolerance and not, for example, shortness of breath that makes him stop walking.

Causes of claudication

1. Atheroma (the commonest cause) leading to narrowing (stenosis), thrombosis or embolism.
2. Buerger's disease (rare).

Claudication is made worse by anaemia.

Questions you need to answer by the end of the history and examination

1. Where is the block?

The arterial system lends itself very much to examination. By the end of the history and examination you should be able to determine the site of arterial occlusion. Arterial disease can of course affect any artery in the body but certain arteries are more at risk:

In the abdomen the most vulnerable are the aorta just at and above the bifurcation, the common iliac arteries and the internal iliac arteries. In the lower limb, the artery most commonly affected is the superficial femoral.

The pain is always in the muscle segment beyond the blockage: thus, if blockage is in the aorta, the pain is in the buttocks; in the iliacs the thigh; and in the superficial femoral artery the calf.

Thus, if the patient presents with whole leg claudication and is found to have a reduced femoral pulse on the affected side, he probably has an aorto-iliac or common iliac occlusion on that side. If he presents with calf claudication and has a normal femoral pulse but absent popliteal and ankle pulses, the block is most likely to be in the superficial femoral artery. It is common to have multiple blocks affecting both the aorto-iliac segment and the femoral artery.

2. What is the cause of the occlusion?

Atheroma is the commonest cause of occlusion. Think of Buerger's disease in a young patient (20–30 years) who smokes heavily. People of certain races, especially Jews and Indians, are more likely than others to have Buerger's disease.

It should be possible also to determine causes of atheroma such as hypertension, smoking, and hereditary factors from the clinical history and examination.

Thrombosis and embolism: An artery affected by atheroma often gradually narrows as a result of thickening of the intima by plaques. If a patient with previously stable or slowly progressive claudication presents with sudden deterioration of symptoms in the limbs, suspect thrombosis or embolism. Thrombosis occurs at the site of existing atheroma. Fragments from a thrombus migrate as emboli and occlude the vessel distally. Emboli from other sources, such as the left atrium in mitral valve disease and atrial fibrillation, can lodge in a vessel already narrowed by atheroma.

Whether an embolus produces symptoms depends on the capacity for collateral vessels to develop to take blood around the point of obstruction. If the vessel is previously occluded by atheroma, the risk of severe ischaemia is greater when an embolus occurs.

Aneurysms: Degeneration of the media of arteries affected by atheroma is the main cause of aneurysms but there is also a familial component. The commonest sites of aneurysms are the infrarenal aorta; the popliteal arteries; the visceral arteries: splenic, renal and coeliac; and the common femoral arteries. The main complication of aneurysm is rupture but occasionally they may obstruct the branches of adjacent vessels, resulting in acute ischaemia. Embolism is another complication of abdominal aortic aneurysm.

Arterial trauma: Injury to an artery can cause acute ischaemia to the parts supplied. The effects are more serious if the artery is compromised by existing disease.

3. Are there any aggravating factors?

Factors such as anaemia, polycythaemia, heart failure, and obesity are important. They make claudication worse: in the case of the first three, there is poor oxygen carriage to the tissues of the lower limb and in the last the excess fat imposes extra work on the heart. Cigarette smoking is a common aggravating factor.

4. How severe is the impairment of arterial flow to the leg?

The claudication distance is a reasonable measure of the amount of blood reaching the lower limb. The presence of rest pain, gangrene, and ulceration indicate severe impairment. Other useful but less precise signs are capillary refilling time and the colour of the limb.

5. How severely is the arterial disease interfering with the patient's life?

The social history is of enormous value here. The answer to this question determines the need for further investigations (especially arteriography) and operation. Thus, a retired watchmaker of 84 who does not do much walking may not find claudication appearing at 500 yards incapacitating, as long as the limb is in no danger; whereas a postman of 55 who has claudication at one-quarter of a mile may have to give up his job.

History

Reason for question	Questions asked	Comment
Find out about onset and progression of claudication	When last could you walk without any pain? When you first started experiencing pain, how far could you walk before pain came on, on the level, uphill, up stairs?	
	Has this distance remained the same, increased, or decreased, and by how much?	An increase occurs in a third of patients and is probably due to the establishment of collateral circulation. Rapidly decreasing claudication distance means diminishing blood supply to the limb; think of the possibility of thrombosis or embolism, aneurysm and trauma
Determine severity of disease	Is the pain associated with numbness and pins and needles?	These symptoms are due to diversion of blood from the skin to muscle: the skin is at risk of ulceration and gangrene
	Have you had pain in the foot and toes while you are resting and not exercising?	This is ischaemic rest pain. It occurs because the blood supply to the limb is not enough to remove the metabolites produced by the tissues even at rest

	What do you do to ease this pain?	The patient tries to ease ischaemic rest pain by hanging the leg down, especially at night
	Have you had any ulcers or sores on your leg? Have you had any black patches on your feet?	Ulcers and gangrene are dangerous. Oxygen supply to the limb is now insufficient to keep the tissues alive
	In a patient with rest pain, ask about paralysis	Enquire about symptoms of acute ischaemia: pain, paraesthesiae, paralysis, 'perishing with cold'. The signs are pallor and pulselessness
Attempt to locate the level of the block	Please can you show me where you get the pain?	The more proximal the block, the higher the level affected by claudication and the more widespread the pain in the limb. Aortic occlusion causes claudication in both limbs. As a rough guide, occlusion in the iliac arteries and above causes pain in the buttock, thigh and calf. Occlusion of the superficial femoral artery produces calf pain
	In men, is there impotence or failure to achieve an erection?	Obstruction of both internal iliac arteries (e.g. aortic occlusion without adequate collateral flow, or atheroma in both internal iliac arteries) causes impotence. This combination of claudication and impotence constitutes the Leriche syndrome

229

Reason for question	Questions asked	Comment
Find out if there are other arteries affected by atheroma	Do you get pain in your chest or shortness of breath when you walk? Have you suffered a heart attack or coronary thrombosis in the past?	Think of angina pectoris due to coronary atheroma. Described more fully under ROS (CVS)
	Do you get any fits, faints or blackouts? Or have you ever had a stroke resulting in weakness of the arms or the legs etc.?	Cerebral atherosclerosis (more fully under ROS (CNS))
	Any abdominal pain during and following meals?	This suggests ischaemia of the bowel due to mesenteric artery occlusion, but may be due to peptic ulcer
Possible causes of atheroma	History of smoking Family history of arterial disease History of hypertension History of diabetes History of raised blood cholesterol	Elaborate on these later in the appropriate sections
ROS	Finish rest of *CVS*, GUS, GIT, *CNS*, and RS	
PMH	See above: hypertension, myocardial infarction, cerebrovascular accident, diabetes, raised blood cholesterol	

FH	Note the family history. In particular any deaths from cardiac infarction, cerebrovascular disease, diabetes. Family history of raised blood cholesterol. Deaths in young members of the family for no apparent reason	Family history is important in all forms of vascular disease
SOCIAL HISTORY		
How does claudication affect his life?	Find out about his occupation, his hobbies etc. It may be useful to record his activities in a typical week. Is his work sedentary (e.g. office work) or one which involves a lot of walking (e.g. postman)? Is he the breadwinner? How many dependants? Where does patient live – ground floor, or high-rise block? How close are shops and other amenities? Does he own a car?	This information is important and will be taken into account when deciding on treatment in an individual patient
	Find out about smoking, and in particular the patient's willingness to cut down or stop	Patients who continue to smoke get poor results from arterial surgery. Patients with Buerger's disease who continue to smoke have a poor prognosis
DRUGS	Hypotensive drugs, especially beta-blockers; other cardiovascular, antidiabetic drugs; lipid lowering drugs; drugs given to improve blood flow for instance naftidrofuryl oxalate (Praxilene)	They are used in arterial disease. Beta-blockers may reduce blood flow in the periphery and therefore make claudication worse
ALLERGIES		

Examination

Reason for examination	Sign elicited	Comment
General well being, clues about predisposing and aggravating factors	Patients with arterial disorder are often well. If patient is ill, think of a coexisting disease such as heart or liver failure. Obesity makes claudication worse, as it increases demand on the myocardium.	
	Look for anaemia or polycythaemia; the latter gives the patient a ruddy complexion. Both aggravate arterial disease: in anaemia there is poor oxygen carrying capacity; in polycythaemia, blood is too viscous to flow in small vessels.	
	Corneal arcus (white ring at junction between iris and sclera)	Common in old people but when it occurs in a young person it may be due to raised blood lipoproteins
	Xanthomata (yellow deposits of lipids under the skin, often of the upper eyelids)	This is suggestive of raised blood lipids
	Nicotine stained fingers	Due to heavy smoking
RS		
CVS	Blood pressure in both arms	A marked difference suggests subclavian artery occlusion

Pulse rate, rhythm, state of arterial wall: start from radial.

At this stage palpate other pulses superior to the thoracic aorta: Ulnar, brachial, axillary, carotid. Listen for carotid bruit

Risk of arterial embolism with atrial fibrillation

Asymptomatic carotid stenosis common in patients with claudication and carries risk of cerebrovascular accident. Note, however, that a carotid bruit does not mean there is carotid stenosis, merely turbulent flow in the vessel

JVP, apex beat, thrills, heart sounds, cardiac murmurs, and other added sounds. Any signs of heart failure

Heart failure aggravates claudication. It may also mask the extent of claudication as the patient will stop walking early because of shortness of breath

ABDOMEN

Evidence of arterial disease and heart failure

Inspection: Scars, for instance from previous arterial operations and sympathectomy

Pulsatile masses

Palpation: Masses with expansile pulsation

May be an aneurysm. An aneurysm causes damage by direct occlusion of blood flow or by emboli from the aneurysm to the arteries distal to it. In very slim patients, aortic pulsation may be very prominent

Enlarged liver with tender edge and venous pulsation

This suggests congestive cardiac failure

Feel for common iliac and external iliac arteries

This is possible especially in slim patients

Auscultation: Bruits over stenosed arteries

They indicate turbulent flow in the affected vessel

233

Reason for examination	Sign elicited	Comment
LOWER LIMBS Assess blood flow to the lower limb. Always compare with the opposite limb	*Inspection:* Colour of the limb	It may be pale or cyanosed when ischaemia is present
	Elevate ⎫ the leg and watch the Depress ⎭ colour	The severely ischaemic leg becomes pale on elevation and blue on depression. This is Buerger's test
	Then hang the leg over the side of the bed and see how long it takes for the leg to become pink again	The longer the time the more severe the ischaemia
	Trophic changes, muscle wasting, ulcers, gangrene	These indicate severe ischaemia
	Oedema of the leg	This may be due to heart failure and is not usually a feature of ischaemia. Venous disease can also coexist
	Palpation: Feel the temperature of both legs. Measure capillary refilling by pressing on the pulp of the toe and blanching it and seeing how long it takes to become pink again. Do this first on the normal limb or on yourself to compare	The longer the capillary refilling time the more severe the occlusion

Feel the femoral, popliteal, posterior
tibial and dorsalis pedis pulses on
both sides and chart. Note the
state of the artery wall

Auscultation: Listen for bruits

Finish rest of abdominal examination, examine
genitalia and do a rectal examination

CNS Neurological signs such as muscle weakness, increased muscle tone and sensory impairment may be
due to cerebrovascular disease from occlusion of the carotid arteries. Intermittent attacks of
dizziness and fainting without permanent neurological damage may be due to microemboli or
ischaemia of the brain from carotid artery obstruction or from vertebrobasilar ischaemia.

If an ulcer is present on the lower limb in a diabetic patient, it is important to determine whether
or not there is sensory impairment in the affected limb. This has management implications, for
an ischaemic ulcer (due to diminished blood supply) will heal only after the blood supply is
improved with reconstructive surgery, whereas as a neuropathic ulcer improves with local
treatment.

Investigations

Every patient with claudication must have the following tests:

Urinalysis for sugar: Diabetes must be considered.

Hb: It is important to rule out anaemia or polycythaemia.

Plasma viscosity: This is important especially if the
haemoglobin is raised. It is a measure of how viscid
the blood is, and is determined by various factors such

as the concentration of plasma proteins and the numbers of red cells. Many laboratories will measure plasma viscosity if requested.

Blood sugar: Diabetes must be excluded in all patients.

ECG: It is important to determine whether the coronary arteries are also occluded by atheroma.

Chest X-ray: Look at the size of the heart, look for calcification of the heart valves and of the aorta, and at the lung fields for evidence of heart failure.

Fasting blood cholesterol: This is especially important in young patients with arterial disease, or where there is a positive family history.

Doppler blood pressure measurement: This method is of great value because it is non-invasive and gives consistently reproducible results. Doppler is simply a device with a probe that detects blood flow. The following are some of its uses:

(a) Detection of arteries which are impalpable: Using the probe it is possible to detect most of the arteries which cannot be felt. The frequency of the sound emitted gives an indication of the speed of flow within the vessel.

(b) Pressure index: In the normal individual the systolic blood pressure at the ankle is greater than that in the brachial artery because of the extra hydrostatic pressure exerted by the column of blood in the leg. The systolic blood pressure can be measured in much the same way as can blood pressure in the arm. A sphygmomanometer cuff is used but the Doppler is the 'listening' device rather than a stethoscope. If the systolic pressure in the leg is divided by that in the arm, the ratio should therefore greater than 1. This ratio is referred to as the pressure index or ankle/brachial index (ABI). Assuming that there is no obstruction to blood flow in the arm, the value of the pressure index correlates fairly well with the degree of impairment of blood flow in the leg. Thus a pressure index between 0.5 and 0.9 indicates intermittent claudication, 0.3–0.5 rest pain, and below this value impending gangrene. The treadmill test is more accurate than a single measure of pressure index at rest.

(c) Treadmill: This is a mechanically operated platform on which a patient walks; its speed and gradient can be altered when necessary. Using this device the distance the patient is able to walk can be accurately calculated and any symptoms associated with claudication, such as shortness of breath or chest pain, can be documented. Pressure index is obtained before exercise and following exercise until it returns to normal. The extent to which the pressure index falls and the time it takes to return to normal are both of great value in determining the degree of impairment. The test can be repeated after reconstructive operations to see if improvement has occurred; it can also be used to monitor the progress of patients who are being followed up in the outpatient clinic. This facility is not available to all vascular surgeons.

Duplex imaging: Duplex imaging, an accurate and non-invasive method of arterial investigation, combines two techniques, hence the name. These are ultrasound, which gives information about the anatomy of the artery (size, presence of stenosis) and a Doppler probe, which tells us about blood flow in the vessel (flow rate, pulse wave, turbulence).

Arteriography: This is an invasive and potentially risky procedure and must not be performed routinely. It is done only in those in whom a reconstructive operation will be performed if the lesion demonstrated is operable. The patient's fitness for such an operation should have been determined before, not after, arteriography. Another value is that therapeutic interventional radiology procedures such as angioplasty or stenting can be performed in suitable cases.

Case report

Features	Analysis
Frank Sturrock is a 66-year-old retired postman. He is caucasian. He is married and lives with his wife on the 6th floor of a block of council flats. He presented to his GP complaining that for the last 18 months he had had pain in his right thigh and calf on walking.	The most common cause of pain on walking at this age is arterial obstruction. Less common causes are spinal canal stenosis and cauda equina lesions, but history will help determine whether we are dealing with intermittent claudication.
He had worked successfully as a postman for most of his life. Before his symptoms started he walked up to 5 kilometres a day, 6 days a week delivering letters from door to door. Six months before he retired he noticed that when he walked about 1 kilometre on the level, he had pain in his right thigh and calf. He had to stop for 4 or 5 minutes and could walk the same distance again before the pain recurred. As this pain did not interfere significantly with his work, he did not consult his GP about it.	This is intermittent claudication. It is common for patients not to complain until the pain begins to interfere with their activities.
When he retired, he did not have to walk as far and did not get much pain. However, over the last 5 months the pain started again but this time came on after he walked 200 metres on the level. By the time he presented, he could walk for only 100 metres. The pain was still in his right thigh and calf and improved after he stopped and rested for about 6 minutes.	The claudication distance has decreased. This suggests that the occlusion has become worse or collateral vessels have become compromised by disease such as extension of atherosclerosis or embolism.

He denied pain at rest and was never woken from sleep with this pain. He did not have any sores or black patches on his legs or feet.

The absence of rest pain is encouraging. Rest pain is due to severe ischaemia.

On direct questioning, he admitted that for the last 2 years, he had rarely attempted sexual intercourse because he could not achieve an erection. This caused marital disharmony and made him depressed.

This is the Leriche syndrome, described above. Patients are often reluctant to present with this distressing symptom and will not talk about it unless asked.

He denied ever having chest pain, undue shortness of breath, fits, faints, blackouts or stroke. He had no pain on eating. There were no other symptoms on review of systems.

Arterial disease is a generalized condition, but it is common for patients to present with symptoms due to disease in one artery. Every attempt must be made to uncover disease in other arteries, especially the coronary, carotid, mesenteric and renal arteries.

He has smoked 35 cigarettes a day since he was 16 years of age and he drank 14 units of alcohol a week. He was diagnosed as hypertensive 10 years ago and has been on a variety of hypotensive drugs. At the time he was taking bendrofluazide 2.5 mg daily. He was not taking any other medications. His GP had told him on numerous occasions that he was overweight and had tried to help him lose weight, but unsuccessfully. He was not known to have diabetes.

Two important risk factors for vascular disease in this patient are smoking and hypertension. His obesity also aggravates his symptoms as the oxygen available is used to move a large body mass.
Note that bendrofluazide has been reported to cause impotence.

His father died from myocardial infarction at the age of 63 and his mother died aged 92 from 'old age'. As far as he knew, no other diseases ran in his family.

Death of a parent or sibling from ischaemic heart is a significant risk factor for coronary heart disease.

Features	Analysis
As mentioned above, Mr Sturrock lives in a block of flats with his wife. They do not own a car but manage to do most of their shopping in a mall near their home. He loved taking long walks in the country at weekends but had to give this up because of the pain in his right leg.	Their essential needs are well catered for despite his disabilities, but he has had to give up an important hobby.
On examination he was well but overweight: his weight was 89 kg and height 1.68 metres. He was not anaemic or cyanosed. There were no signs of raised blood lipids such as xanthomata, but his fingers were heavily nicotine stained.	Obesity confirmed. Nicotine stained fingers are further evidence of heavy smoking.
BP was 150/95 in both arms, and pulse 84/min and regular. The arteries felt thicker than normal. The ulnar, radial, brachial, axillary and carotid pulses were all present. There were no carotid bruits. Examination of the heart and lungs did not reveal any abnormalities.	This level of blood pressure is acceptable in an obese man of this age. It is important to do a thorough cardiovascular examination in all patients suspected of having vascular disease.
The abdomen was not distended and had no scars, dilated veins or pulsatile masses. The liver, kidneys and spleen were not palpable. The aorta was difficult to palpate, owing to the patient's obesity. On auscultation, a bruit was audible in the right lower quadrant just above the inguinal ligament.	Bruits are due to turbulent flow in stenosed arteries. The vessels to think of in this case are the right common iliac, and renal and mesenteric arteries.

The lower limbs were next examined and the two sides compared. The colour was normal and there was no oedema or varicose veins. There was no change in colour on elevation or depression of the limbs. There were no trophic changes, muscle wasting, ulcers or gangrene.

Examination of the lower limbs is most important. The two sides must be compared, as it is easy otherwise to miss subtle abnormalities.

The right lower limb felt cooler than the left, especially below the knee. Capillary refilling time was the same in both legs. The pulses on the left were all present and normal. On the right, the femoral pulse was weak and the pulses below this point were absent. The bruit heard in the abdomen was described above.

There are definite abnormalities on the right. In the presence of a weak femoral pulse and a bruit in the lower abdomen on the same side, the most likely site of stenosis is the right common iliac artery. External iliac disease occurs but is much less common. The significance of his impotence in relation to the site of arterial block is discussed below.

Rectal examination showed a slightly enlarged, benign prostate and no other abnormalities. The locomotor and neurological systems were normal.

Although there is nothing to suggest locomotor disturbance, it is useful to examine this system fully.

Clinical diagnosis
As discussed above, we now need to answer five questions as follows:

1. Where is the block? Claudication in the thigh and calf suggests a high lesion (above the inguinal ligament), and this is confirmed by the reduction in the volume of the right femoral pulse. The commonest site of a unilateral stenosis above the inguinal ligament is the common iliac artery. The external iliac artery can be affected but much less commonly. How does the impotence fit into this picture? It may be unrelated and psychogenic in cause, or it may be due to bendrofluazide. If it is due to reduced blood flow to the erectile tissues of the penis, as seems likely from the nature of the impotence, its cause is obstruction of both internal iliac arteries. As the blood flow to the left lower limb is normal, we have to postulate an

| *Features* | *Analysis* |

isolated block in the left internal iliac artery. Some blood is getting through the right common and external iliac arteries but perhaps not enough to perfuse the right internal iliac; or there may be an additional block in the right internal iliac artery.

2. What is the cause of the occlusion? Atheroma is the most likely cause in this man. From his age, race and the asymmetrical nature of his disease, atheroma is the commonest cause of occlusion. Buerger's disease, the other cause of arterial occlusion, is most unlikely in this man. There is no suggestion of an aneurysm or embolism from a proximal thrombus.

3. Are there any aggravating factors? The most important in this man is obesity.

4. How severe is the impairment of arterial flow to the leg? The claudication distance has diminished rapidly over about 5 months. This is significant and implies further decrease in the calibre of the vessel at the site of occlusion or reduction in blood flow through collateral vessels from involvement by atherosclerosis.

5. How severely is the arterial disease interfering with the patient's life? This man has given up walking because of his arterial disease, but other social needs are met. His impotence has caused marked impairment of the quality of his life.

Investigations

There was no glucose or protein in the urine on analysis.
Hb, plasma viscosity, U&Es, LFTs and blood glucose were normal.

The patient was not diabetic and did not have anaemia or polycythaemia. An impairment of U&Es in this man would suggest renal involvement from hypertension or atherosclerosis of the renal arteries.

There were no changes on ECG to suggest ischaemia or ventricular hypertrophy.
Chest X-ray was normal.
Fasting blood lipids were normal.

A normal resting ECG should not be taken as evidence of absence of coronary disease. Even an exercise ECG is of limited value because this man's claudication may prevent him from walking far enough to get chest pain.

Doppler blood flow measurements:

The ankle-brachial systolic pressure index on the left was 0.9 and on the right 0.6.

Exercise on the treadmill confirmed claudication occurred at 150 metres on the level. The pre-exercise pressure index on the right was 0.6. It dropped to 0.03 when his claudication developed and took 12 minutes to return to the resting value.

A resting pressure index of 0.6 indicates severe claudication. The treadmill test is more useful and shows severe ischaemia of the right lower limb on exercise.

Final diagnosis

A decision was made that this patient needed reconstructive arterial surgery. This was because of the rapidly diminishing claudication distance and the critically low pressure index. He was advised to stop smoking and to lose weight. Arteriography showed severe stenosis of the right common iliac artery at its origin from the aorta, but there was good flow in the superficial femoral and distal vessels through collaterals. There was little flow in the right internal iliac artery and a complete block of the left internal iliac artery.

Chapter 16

Venous disorders of the lower limbs

While the arterial system supplies blood to the lower limb to provide for the metabolic needs of the tissues not only at rest but also during exercise, the venous system drains deoxygenated blood and toxic metabolites rapidly and completely. Failure of adequate venous drainage (venous insufficiency) can occur if (a) the vein or veins are obstructed or (b) if the valves which normally ensure that blood flows in one direction only (viz towards the heart) are incompetent.

Possible sites affected by venous disorders of the lower limb

Venous disorders can affect one or more of the following venous systems.

1. GREAT AND SMALL SAPHENOUS VEINS AND THEIR BRANCHES: The veins are superficial to the deep fascia of the lower limb and are therefore visible and/or palpable when they dilate. Dilatation of these veins is commonly due to incompetence of the venous valves: the sapheno-femoral, the sapheno-popliteal, and the perforating vein valves. Valves can become incompetent for no demonstrable reason or following thrombosis. Patients under the age of 25 years with varicose veins give a positive family history in 75% of cases. This suggests a hereditary venous valve defect. There is a familial incidence in 40% of all cases of varicose veins.

2. FEMORAL AND POPLITEAL VEINS: These can be occluded by a thrombus. Thrombosis can occur during operations or because of prolonged immobility. They can be occluded by malignancy (e.g. lymph nodes infiltrated by malignancy) or damaged by operation or irradiation.

3. COMMON ILIAC OR EXTERNAL ILIAC VEINS: These can be occluded by thrombus,

embolus, or can be accidentally damaged during pelvic operations. They can also be obstructed by pressure from outside the wall, for instance by pelvic 'tumours' such as the pregnant uterus, fibroids, and malignant tumours of the gynaecological organs. Iliac vein thrombosis is common after orthopaedic, gynaecological and other operations in and around the pelvis.

4. INFERIOR VENA CAVA: This can be occluded by thrombus, by infected embolus, or by surgical ligation to prevent pulmonary embolism.

Systemic or remote factors that predispose to venous thrombosis include:

1. The oral contraceptive pill.
2. Malignant disease, especially of the pancreas.
3. Prolonged immobilization.
4. Abnormalities of the clotting system, for instance thrombocytosis, polycythaemia rubra vera.
5. Following operations, especially on the hips and pelvis.

There are four important consequences of venous insufficiency:

1. Varicose veins.
2. Swelling of the leg.
3. Ulceration.
4. Other skin changes such as eczema and pigmentation.

It is important to remember that varicose veins are only one consequence of venous insufficiency; they may be absent in the more severe cases of venous insufficiency. The term 'varicose ulcer' is therefore regarded by some as incorrect; 'venous ulcer' is more apt. Others prefer the term 'gravitational' ulcer.

When attempting to make a diagnosis in a patient with venous insufficiency, the student has four tasks:

1. To determine what systemic causes may be present.
2. To determine what local causes are present, i.e. occlusion or valvular incompetence.
3. To determine the veins which are involved, e.g. inferior vena cava, iliac veins, femoral or popliteal veins, or the great or small saphenous veins and their branches.

4. To determine the consequences of venous insufficiency, namely varicose veins, ulceration, etc.

Presenting complaint(s)

The common presenting complaints of venous disorders of the lower limb are:

1. Varicose veins, i.e. presenting as a cosmetic problem initially but later causing some of the symptoms in 2. below.
2. Pain or discomfort in the legs, heaviness of the legs, irritation or itching.
3. Ulcers.
4. Swelling of the legs.
5. Other skin changes such as stasis pigmentation.

Points to look for

1. Any systemic disease present such as polycythaemia or malignancy? A ruddy complexion suggests polycythaemia; weight loss, malaise, anaemia, lymphadenopathy and abdominal masses should raise the suspicion of malignancy, but these signs may be absent in many patients with cancer.
2. Which veins are involved? Dilated, tortuous veins on the abdominal wall suggest occlusion of the inferior vena cava. Occlusion of the iliac veins should be suspected if there has been previous pelvic surgery, pelvic irradiation, or the white leg of pregnancy. A history of deep venous thrombosis suggests iliac, femoral or popliteal vein thrombosis.

   Marked skin changes at the ankle, namely ulceration, eczema, pigmentation and oedema, especially in the presence of significant varicose veins, are either due to occlusion of the deep veins (iliac, femoral, or popliteal), or to the presence of local incompetent perforating veins around the ankle.

   If the patient presents with asymptomatic varicose veins, or where the symptoms are minimal, the diagnosis is most often primary varicose veins or secondary varicose veins due to valvular destruction.

3. What is the main consequence of venous insufficiency? Is it varicose veins, venous ulceration or other skin disorder, or oedema? This should be clear from the history.

History

Reason for question	Question asked	Comment
Which of the complaints listed above bothers the patient most	*Varicose veins:* How long have they been present? Are they getting worse or have they stayed the same over the past months or years? Please show me where the veins are that bother you One leg or both?	
	What is it that concerns you most about these veins? (Let the patient tell you about his concerns in his own words; then:) Is it they way they look, are they unsightly? (i.e. cosmetic) Or are they causing any symptoms such as pain discomfort etc. (i.e. symptomatic) see below	

Reason for question	Question asked	Comment
	Symptoms: Please can you describe to me the pain you get?	The pain is usually described as a dull ache
	Where is the pain or the discomfort?	It is located in the calves or occasionally around the ankle
	At what time of day is the pain worst?	Pain from varicose veins is worst at the end of the day when the patient has been on his feet, and gets better if he puts his feet up or lies down. Some patients also get cramp in the calf at night
	What makes the pain better?	
	Do you get any pain when you walk?	Patients with venous insufficiency sometimes get a tearing pain in the calf when they walk. This pain is sometimes referred to as *venous claudication*
	Any other symptoms such as heaviness of the legs or itching?	These are sometimes reported
	Do your feet and legs swell? If so, when?	Swelling due to varicose veins is worst at the end of the day. If the swelling is present all the time, severe venous insufficiency is probably present
	Ulcer (if present): When did the ulcer first appear?	
	What caused it?	Often trivial trauma
	How has it progressed since?	It takes a long time to heal, or it may heal only to break down again

What was the state of the skin before the ulcer started?

Usually the skin is unhealthy and may have been pigmented or had eczema

Swelling: Where is the swelling?
How bad does it get?
When does it occur?

Swelling of the ankle with varicose veins is mild and occurs at the end of the day when the patient has been on his feet. If the swelling is present all the time, think of the possibility of venous insufficiency. If the swelling is bilateral, consider other causes such as heart failure and hypoproteinaemia

Other skin changes: Has there been darkening of the skin, weeping, a rash?

Hyperpigmentation and eczema are common with venous insufficiency

Has the skin broken down into an ulcer?

Poor skin nutrition leads to ulceration. The skin changes of chronic venous insufficiency are referred to as *lipodermatosclerosis*. The features are redness or blackness of the skin, pitting oedema, thickening and tenderness

ROS

CVS: Enquire especially about intermittent claudication, as arterial insufficiency can co-exist with venous disorder. Moreover, congestive cardiac failure resulting in lower limb oedema will impair venous return and aggravate the effects of venous disease.

RS, GUS, CNS, GIT

Reason for question	Question asked	Comment
PMH	Past history of deep venous thrombosis, pelvic operations, pelvic irradiation	
	In a woman, history of pregnancy, varicose veins first appearing during pregnancy, swollen leg during pregnancy	Most varicose veins appearing during pregnancy subside a few weeks after delivery. They are due to pressure on the pelvic veins by the enlarged uterus, and to some extent the dilatory effect of progesterone on smooth muscle. In some women the veins persist
	History of fibroids?	They can press on pelvic veins and raise venous pressure in the lower limbs
FH	Any family history of varicose veins?	A positive history can be elicited in a 40% of patients. In those under 25 years, this figure is higher
SH	Occupation: does this involve the patient standing in one place for a long time? Does it involve heavy lifting?	The symptoms of varicose veins are aggravated by these factors
	Smoking	This increases the risk of venous thrombosis
DRUGS	Oral contraceptive pill	Increased risk of venous thrombosis especially in women who smoke
ALLERGIES		

Examination

Reason for examination	Sign elicited	Comment
General examination	Patients with venous disease are well. If ill, consider coexisting disease such as malignancy. Some are obese.	
Systematic exam	RS, CVS, CNS	
Consider lesions that impede or occlude venous return	Abdominal masses Any dilated veins across the abdominal wall?	Suggesting inferior vena caval obstruction
	In women, do vaginal examination. Rectal examination in both sexes Examine the genitalia	It is not always practical or desirable to perform pelvic examination in every patient with varicose veins
LOWER LIMBS	*Inspection:* Stand the patient up and examine from groin down to toes. Examine front, backs and sides of both limbs	
	If varicose veins present, record their anatomical distribution and size	Varicose veins on the medial side of the leg may extend from the groin to the calf
	Start from the groins, look for saphena varix Look for scars of previous varicose veins operations	They are due to dilatation of the great saphenous vein and its branches
	Look for vulval or scrotal varicosities Note any telangiectasia: these are fine spidery veins	Varicose veins on the back of the calf from the knee down are dilatations of the small saphenous vein and its tributaries

251

Reason for examination	Sign elicited	Comment
	Note the relation of any veins to the great and small saphenous veins	A varicosity may extend from the medial side of the thigh downwards and laterally to the knee and end on the lateral side of the calf. It is the lateral superficial femoral vein – a branch of the great saphenous vein
	Inspect the skin: Any pigmentation, ulceration or eczema?	
	If an ulcer is found, examine it carefully as previously described. Note any infection in it Examine for inguinal lymph node enlargement	
	Palpation: Thrombosed veins. Thickness of the skin Pitting oedema	Some authorities claim that it is possible by palpation to locate the sites of perforating veins as defects in the deep fascia, but many doubt whether this can be done accurately
	Palpate all varicose veins	Some veins are better felt than seen
	Cough impulse test: Place a finger over the sapheno-femoral junction with patient standing up and ask him to cough	If a thrill is felt down the great saphenous vein it suggests sapheno-femoral incompetence

Percussion test: While the patient is still standing, place two fingers of the left hand over the great saphenous just below the point where it enters the femoral vein. With the middle finger of the right hand, tap over the main varices below on the thigh and note any impulse felt by the left hand

Continue percussing the vein downwards with the right hand until an impulse can no longer be felt by the left hand

If valves in the segment of vein between the left hand and the right hand are incompetent, or if there are no valves between the two points, the wave generated by the percussing hand is felt by the palpating hand

Many doubt the accuracy of the cough impulse and percussion tests in detecting saphenofemoral incompetence

The Brodie–Trendelenburg test (Fig 16.1): Lie the patient on his back on the couch. Lift the limb to allow blood to drain completely from the vein(s). If necessary, massage the blood from the toes to the groin with the leg elevated

Place a tourniquet round the thigh distal to the level of the saphenofemoral junction. Ask the patient to stand up

With the tourniquet in place and the patient standing up, the varicose veins will stay collapsed. In this case the incompetence is at the saphenofemoral junction

Now release the tourniquet and watch the veins fill

If the veins fill quickly, the valve is incompetent. This is a positive test

If the tourniquet just below the saphenofemoral junction fails to keep the varicose veins collapsed, repeat the test but place the tourniquet just above the knee

If this tourniquet now succeeds in controlling the veins, the incompetence is in the midthigh region, through a perforator

253

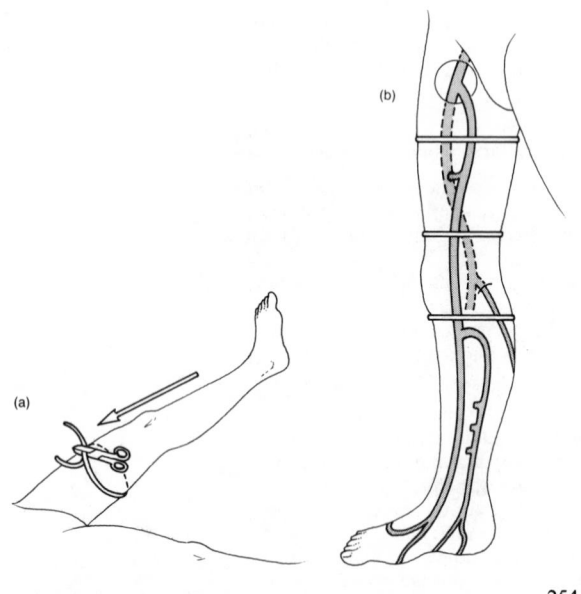

Figure 16.1. *The Brodie–Trendelenburg test. (a) The patient is on his back, the limb is lifted and the blood drained and a tourniquet applied around the upper thigh. (b) By applying the tourniquet at different sites on the thigh and leg in succession it is possible to determine the site of venous incompetence*

Reason for examination	Sign elicited	Comment
	If the small saphenous vein is dilated, repeat the test with the tourniquet around the upper calf just distal to the sapheno-popliteal junction	
	Examine all the pulses in the lower limb	It is important to remember that many elderly patients presenting with venous insufficiency of the lower limb also have arterial disease. Conventional treatment with compression and other measures would clearly be dangerous for such patients
	Auscultation: Listen over dilated veins	Any bruits suggest arterio-venous communications.

Investigations

Many investigations are described for the diagnosis of venous insufficiency but few are used in practice. This underlines the great value of the history and examination. Most patients presenting with uncomplicated varicose veins do not undergo tests.

Hb: This will indicate the presence of anaemia or polycythaemia.

ESR: A raised ESR suggests the presence of malignancy or infection of a venous ulcer.

Doppler ultrasound flow detector: This technique determines back flow at the sapheno-femoral and sapheno-popliteal valves, and also at the sites of suspected perforating veins. Simply place the Doppler probe over the sapheno-femoral. Squeeze the calf and you will hear the sound made by the increase in blood flow towards the heart. With an incompetent system there will also be rapid reflux when the calf is released, giving an abnormal 'back flow' sound.

Phlebography or venography: Is the procedure in which contrast is injected into the vein in order to outline its structure. Injection is into a superficial pedal vein, but this simply outlines the superficial system. For a deep venogram, a venous tourniquet is applied around the calf. Phlebography shows the presence of thrombi and other abnormalities within the vein. Venous collaterals will also be shown as will the presence of perforating veins. It is rarely performed because it is invasive.

Abdominal ultrasound: Is useful in defining the nature of any masses found in the abdomen or in the pelvis during the examination.

Patients with suspected venous ulcers should have non-invasive assessment of the deep veins to determine whether they are (a) patent and (b) competent. This is done with *plethysmography* or *duplex scanning*. Plethysmography assesses changes in the volume of the limb, while duplex scanning (also used in arterial disease) gives information about the anatomy of the veins and the flow of blood through them.

Biopsy of ulcers of uncertain nature: Gravitational or venous ulcers can be easily recognized by their location and their characteristics. If there is any doubt about the nature of an ulcer, a biopsy should be taken to ensure that it is not malignant.

Case report

Features	Analysis
Shirley Brown is aged 25 and works as a shopkeeper. She is married and has one daughter. She saw her GP a few months ago with large veins on her left leg and aching of her left calf and ankle. These symptoms have been more pronounced since her pregnancy 3 years ago.	The diagnosis of varicose veins is usually not in doubt but every attempt must be made to rule out an underlying cause and possible complications. Veins are commoner in women, especially between the ages of 20 and 50. It is common for the symptoms to appear during pregnancy. If veins are present before pregnancy, they are made worse during its progress.

She has always been well and never had any serious illnesses. She was on the oral contraceptive pill from the age of 20 and stopped taking it when she married at the age of 22. A year later she noticed dilated veins on the medial side of her left leg and calf. At first these were small veins. She regarded them merely as a cosmetic blemish and they caused no symptoms.

She became pregnant later that year and found that the veins enlarged as the pregnancy progressed. Her left calf also swelled, especially at the end of the day and the whole leg felt heavy and ached. Her GP prescribed compression stockings, which eased her symptoms considerably. She also felt relief if she put her feet up while she was resting.

After she delivered, the veins got much smaller but never disappeared completely. Over the last 3 years the veins got larger and the symptoms she had during pregnancy returned. She has not noticed any darkening of the skin of her legs, an ulcer or a rash.

There were no other symptoms on systems enquiry. She did not have intermittent claudication or a history of venous thrombosis. She had not undergone any operations and had no major illnesses. She did not go back on the oral contraceptive pill after her delivery. She did not smoke but drank 7 units of alcohol a week. She worked as a shopkeeper 3 days a week to supplement the family income.

Women on the pill have an increased chance of deep venous thrombosis, especially if they smoke. This lady stopped the pill before the veins developed. The initial problem in many is cosmetic, but symptoms develop later.

The symptoms from varicose veins often improve with compression stockings and elevation. This helps to distinguish between the symptoms of venous and arterial disease. The latter are made worse by these two factors.

Varicose veins generally improve after pregnancy, but in some patients, they get worse. She had none of the skin complications described above as ascribed to venous disease.

Arterial disease in unusual at this age but it must always be sought because, as mentioned above, some methods of treatment of venous disease are contraindicated in the presence of arterial disorders. There was no apparent cause for her varicose veins such as pelvic surgery. Her work, involving standing up, does not cause varicose veins, but aggravates the symptoms.

Features	Analysis
Her mother and grandmother had severe varicose veins from an early age. Her mother had several operations for her veins. No one else in the family had venous disorders.	As discussed above, a family history can be elicited in over 40% of patients with varicose veins.
She looked well and was not anaemic. She was moderately obese. There were no abnormalities in her head and neck. Blood pressure and pulse were normal as were the heart and lungs.	Some patients with varicose veins are obese but most are otherwise well.
There were no abnormalities on examination of the abdomen and groins. Rectal and vaginal examination did not reveal any pelvic masses	It is important to rule out pelvic tumours as a cause of varicose veins.
The legs were examined first with the patient standing up. The right leg was normal apart from telangiectasia on the back of the calf. There were no vulval varices or saphena varix. On the right was a dilated vein running from the upper thigh down the medial side to the middle of the calf. There was no skin pigmentation or ulceration. There were telangiectasia on the back of the left calf but no significantly dilated veins on this aspect of the leg.	Telangiectasia are frequently seen on the legs, even in the absence of varicose veins. The varicose vein on the right is running along the course of the great saphenous vein.
The dilated vein on the left could be easily palpated and was tortuous throughout its course. There were several tributaries feeding into it along its length. The vein was not thrombosed and there was no pitting oedema.	Palpation is a useful means of locating varicose veins as some veins are easier to feel than to see.

The patient (still standing) was asked to cough, with the examiner's finger over the left sapheno-femoral junction. A thrill was felt down the great saphenous vein.

This suggests sapheno-femoral incompetence.

The percussion test (see text) was positive along the course of the left great saphenous vein down to the knee. The Brodie–Trendelenburg test (see text) showed sapheno-femoral incompetence. It was not possible to locate the sites of perforating veins.

The interpretation is that the valves along the course of the great saphenous vein are incompetent down to the level of the knee. This is not an accurate test.

There was no evidence of arterial impairment in either leg and all pulses were were present and normal.

As mentioned in the text, you must examine the arterial system in the leg in all patients with varicose veins.

Clinical diagnosis
She has varicose veins affecting the right great saphenous vein. There was sapheno-femoral incompetence and incompetent valves down to the level of the knee. Sapheno-femoral incompetence was confirmed by the Doppler ultrasound flow detector, but no other tests were carried out.

Chapter 17

Head injury

Each year in Britain, almost 1 million patients with head injuries attend hospital. Of these, nearly 155 000 are admitted, 5000 die and 1000, most of whom are young men, survive with severe disabilities. This largely preventable problem is an important cause of morbidity and mortality.

Aims of head injury management

The role of general surgeons in head injury management is an important one, but one about which there is much confusion. The detection of the relatively few patients who need to be transferred for specialist neurosurgical care, though important, is only a small part of the overall responsibility. The aims of head injury management are as follows:

1. To save life. Many patients die not from the injury to the brain, but from avoidable factors such as inhalation of vomit and other causes of acute airway obstruction. A much smaller number die from complications of the head injury such as subdural haematoma.

2. To prevent secondary brain damage. There are two types of brain damage.
   (a) Primary brain damage. This is damage due directly to the injury itself. Unfortunately brain tissue does not regenerate and, once structural damage has occurred, the dead tissue will be replaced by glial scar tissue (gliosis). The brain has a fairly good reserve functional capacity, and it is therefore possible to retrain the viable parts to restore some of the functions of those parts that are lost.
   (b) Secondary brain damage. This is further damage to an already injured brain, and is caused by factors which include the following:
      i. Hypoxia, for instance, from shock, respiratory obstruction or lung damage.

ii. Infections of the brain: meningitis, encephalitis, cerebral abscess. These are particularly likely after open skull injury.
iii. Acid-base disturbance.
iv. Hypoglycaemia.
v. Hyperpyrexia.
vi. Compression of brain tissue due to subdural, extradural and intracerebral haematoma; depressed skull fracture; cerebral oedema.

Whereas primary brain damage cannot be prevented (except by preventing the accident or reducing the impact to the brain), secondary brain damage is largely preventable.

3. To treat associated injuries in order of seriousness. Thus, whatever the severity of brain damage, if the spleen has also been ruptured, laparotomy must be performed and the bleeding stopped. On the other hand, an uncomplicated fracture of a long bone can await definitive treatment for several hours until the patient's condition has stabilized.

4. To prevent or reduce the disabilities due to the injury, for example traumatic epilepsy, or those due to immobilization such as pressure sores and muscle contractures.
5. To treat symptoms such as pain and to provide psychological support.
6. To rehabilitate the patient.

The comatose patient who has sustained a head injury

A lot of time is often lost doing inappropriate investigations on patients who sustain a head injury before developing coma. The head injury may be minor but it is presumed to be the cause of the loss of consciousness. This delays recognition of the underlying disorder. Some important causes of coma are disease of the central nervous system such as meningitis, subarachnoid haemorrhage and cerebrovascular accident, alcohol, drugs, hypoglycaemia and hyperglycaemia, uraemia and epilepsy.

The following is an account of the principles of diagnosis and initial management of patients in the first few hours after head injury.

Unless special equipment is available the following should be done.

1. Clear airway; give mouth-to-mouth respiration if necessary. *Care in handling the neck:* the cervical spine may be fractured. It is safer to assume that the cervical spine has been fractured, until proved otherwise. A cervical collar, if available, should be applied routinely.
2. Apply pressure to bleeding wounds.
3. Gently splint limbs which may be fractured.
4. Call for an ambulance.
5. If the patient is conscious, explain to him what has happened and reassure.
6. Make a mental note of the patient's level of consciousness and note the size of the pupils (see below).

On arrival in the accident department

The patient must be carefully but swiftly moved from the ambulance to the emergency room. Again, the neck must be handled carefully. The neck is stabilized with a cervical collar, if this has not been applied already.

Baseline observations (see later in text)

Primary survey and resuscitation

Even if the patient's condition appears satisfactory, you must go through again the routine for emergency care, checking the airway, breathing and circulation, and resuscitate if necessary. If resuscitation is unnecessary, or if following resuscitation the patient's condition is now stable, a full history is taken and a thorough examination performed.

If resuscitation is necessary because the patient is not breathing well or is shocked, it is important to answer certain questions:

Have normal respirations been established?

Signs such as respiratory distress, shallow and laboured respirations, cyanosis and stridor may be due to obstruction of the airway. Common causes of airway obstruction are blood, vomit, dentures and tissue damage due to direct trauma to the upper airway. If after adequate clearance of the airway there is no improvement in respiration, the patient should be intubated and ventilated.

Has the patient responded to adequate fluid infusion?

1. Yes. Sometimes the patient will be shocked because he lost a lot of blood from superficial wounds such as those on the scalp. If there is no current bleeding, the patient should respond well to adequate infusion. If you are satisfied that he is no longer shocked, proceed to take the history.
2. No. If a patient remains in shock in spite of adequate fluid replacement, he is probably still bleeding from somewhere else. *It must be emphasized that it is unusual to get shock due entirely to head injury.* If there is no external bleeding, then internal haemorrhage must be suspected. Common internal sources of bleeding include damaged spleen, liver, kidney and great vessels. In such a case, it is

important to insert a central venous cannula and to monitor central venous pressure (CVP). It would be wise also to insert a urinary catheter to monitor urinary output, but urethral injury must be excluded (see below).

If the answer to the above question is no, where is the bleeding occurring?

1. The chest: do an urgent portable chest X-ray. This will confirm the position of the CVP line and may give an indication of the source of bleeding: if there is no pleural effusion or widened mediastinum, then the source of bleeding is almost certainly not in the thoracic cavity.
   (a) Widened mediastinum: this may be due to damage to the thoracic aorta.
   (b) If haemothorax present, a chest drain must be inserted and the amount of blood lost from it carefully monitored and replaced. Thoracotomy may be necessary if the patient is needing more than about one unit of blood each hour to maintain his blood pressure and CVP.

2. The abdomen: abdominal X-ray cannot give useful information about intra-abdominal bleeding. Three methods have been described for determining whether there is free blood in the peritoneal cavity:

(a) Abdominal girth measurements: do not rely on abdominal girth measurements, for they are misleading. The peritoneal cavity may hold up to 3 litres of blood without an increase of abdominal girth. On the other hand, a small amount of retroperitoneal bleeding can cause rapid paralytic ileus and hence an increase in abdominal girth.

(b) Four-quadrant peritoneal aspiration: a needle is inserted into the four quadrants of the peritoneal cavity and the contents aspirated. Assuming that the needle does not cause trauma, any blood, especially old dark blood, is presumed to be lying free in the peritoneal cavity. It is difficult to be sure that blood in the syringe is not from trauma of the procedure, and it is easy to get a dry tap even when there is a lot of blood in the peritoneal cavity.

(c) Peritoneal lavage: a catheter is inserted into the peritoneal cavity and saline infused. The fluid is drained after a few minutes and inspected to see how much blood is present in it. The same reservations apply to this method as to b. above, but performed carefully, it gives accurate information about bleeding in the peritoneal cavity.

3. Long bone fractures: up to 2 litres of blood can be lost from a fracture of the neck of the femur without much swelling of the surrounding tissues. If a long bone fracture is present, more blood should be given before it is presumed that the patient has not responded.

Is the abdominal cavity a possible source of bleeding?

If there is no haemothorax and bleeding from long bone fracture has been allowed for, then continuing haemorrhage must be presumed to be from the abdominal cavity. If peritoneal lavage is positive, bleeding is certainly from the abdomen. Before laparotomy is performed, an urgent IVU must be done if time permits, for bleeding may be from one kidney. If it is necessary to remove this kidney it is important to make sure that the opposite one is normal. Ultrasound is useful in detecting certain conditions such as rupture of the spleen, if the abdomen is not distended with gas. Six units of blood must be cross matched and the patient prepared for operation.

Baseline observations

Three important groups of observations must be made and recorded as soon as the patient arrives in hospital. It is important for these to be accurate and to be recorded clearly, for the patient's subsequent progress will be judged from them. The three groups of observations are the Glasgow Coma Scale, the patient's vital signs and pupillary reactions. The value of such a scoring system is that even an inexperienced observer will be able to tell whether there is improvement or deterioration.

1. Glasgow Coma Scale

This is taken as the best response in three categories:

eye opening, verbal response and motor response (Hope *et al.,* 1989). Responses obtained from the two sides, if different, can be recorded separately.

	Response	*Score*
Eye opening	Spontaneous	4
	To name	3
	To pain	2
	None	1
Best verbal response	Orientated	5
	Confused	4
	Inappropriate	3
	Incomprehensible	2
	None	1
Best motor response	Obeying	6
	Localizing	5
	Withdrawal	4
	Abnormal flexion	3
	Extension	2
	None	1

The higher the score the better the prognosis; similarly, low scores, particularly if not responding to

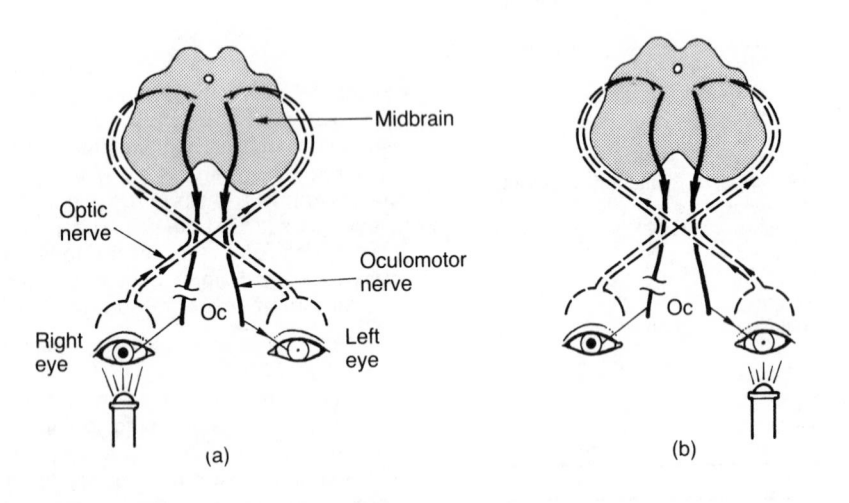

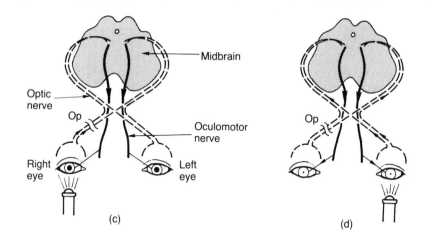

Figure 17.1. *Pupillary reactions to light. Right oculomotor nerve lesion at Oc (for instance by right extradural haematoma). Illuminating the pupil on the right (a) fails to produce constriction of the right pupil, but causes constriction of the left pupil. Illuminating the left pupil (b) produces the same reaction. Right optic nerve lesion at Op (due to direct injury to the eye). Illuminating the right eye fails to constrict both pupils (c), but illuminating the left causes both pupils to constrict (d). Brain compression is likely on one side if the pupil on that side fails to constrict when either pupil is illuminated*

treatment, carry a bad prognosis for the patient. Deterioration after an initially good score is often due to cerebral compression, which is treatable. Death in such a situation is considered to be avoidable.

2. Vital signs

(a) Blood pressure
(b) Pulse
(c) Temperature
(d) Respirations

3. Pupillary reactions

The student often misinterprets these signs because he has not appreciated the basis for them. The afferent or sensory pathway of the pupillary light reflex is carried by the optic nerve to the midbrain. Here it relays with the efferent or motor fibres which are carried in the oculomotor or third cranial nerve. These nerves, when stimulated, constrict the pupil (Fig 17.1). As each optic nerve carries fibres to both parts of the mid-brain, illumination of one eye produces constriction of both pupils. The reaction by the pupil which is illuminated is said to be direct, and that by the opposite pupil consensual. If one cerebral hemisphere is compressed by haematoma, it is the third nerve which, by virtue of its position and course, becomes compressed. The pupil on the affected side dilates because the sympathetic fibres which dilate it are intact and unopposed. When this pupil is illuminated, the direct light reaction will be absent but the consensual reaction will be present. If the pupil on the unaffected side is illuminated, it will constrict but the pupil on the affected side will not. Contrast this with the situation which occurs when the optic nerve is damaged (this damage is due to direct injury to the orbit and does not indicate life-threatening cerebral compression). In this case, when the blind eye is illuminated, its pupil (which is of normal size) will not constrict, nor will the opposite one, because of interruption of the afferent pathways to both pupils. However, if the normal pupil is illuminated, both pupils will constrict. It is clearly important to distinguish between the two conditions by noting the size of the pupils and their reaction to direct and consensual illumination.

History

Take the history from the patient if he is conscious, and also from eye-witnesses, police, ambulance crew, etc.

Reason for question	Questions asked	Comment
Make an accurate note of the times of important events relating to this accident	When did the accident occur? How soon did the ambulance arrive? How long did the journey to the hospital take? When did the patient arrive in the accident department?	These observations may not assist in making an immediate diagnosis but help to give a complete picture of the circumstances of the accident. Any delay in getting help may well account for avoidable complications
Details of accident	Where did the accident occur? If road traffic accident, was the patient a pedestrian, driver or passenger? If he was in a car, was he wearing a seat belt? What were the speeds and directions of the cars at the time of impact?	It is not always possible to get answers to all these questions but an attempt should be made to obtain as much detail as possible of the circumstances of the accident. They may indicate the severity of head and other injuries
	How did the accident happen? What were the sites of impact? How much damage was there to the vehicles? Had any of the drivers and the patient been drinking alcohol or taken illegal drugs?	
	If not a road traffic accident, describe how head injury occurred, noting the forces involved and their speed, direction and sites of impact on the head	

Reason for question	Questions asked	Comment
First aid at the site of the accident	How soon did the police and the ambulance arrive? What first aid was given and with what effect? How much blood was there at the site of the injury?	Effective first aid given at the site of the accident may save the patient's life and reduce the chance of secondary brain damage
Has there been a deterioration in the Glasgow Coma Scale?	What was the patient's Glasgow Coma Scale when help first arrived and thereafter?	Any deterioration since the accident may be due to cerebral compression (see later)
Symptoms accompanying the head injury	Did the patient lose consciousness? For how long?	Transient loss of consciousness may be due to concussion
	Any fits or convulsions?	Convulsions in an epileptic may be the cause of the head injury
	Any headaches, double vision, vomiting, weakness?	Persistent vomiting, especially in children, is an indication for admission and observation
ROS	RS, CVS, CNS, GUS, GIT	A thorough review of systems is important, as it may give an indication of associated injury. For instance abdominal pain and haematuria suggest renal tract injury

PMH, FH, SH,	Assess previous health, occupation, hobbies,
DRUGS,	mood, personality, habits. *Also, past history*
ALLERGIES	*may indicate why head injury occurred, e.g.*
	epilepsy, cerebrovascular accident, drug
	overdoses or diabetes

Examination

Reason for examination	*Sign elicited*	*Comment*
General examination	Look for signs of injury and shock. These include an ill looking patient, anaemia or pallor, cyanosis; signs of shock include a cold periphery and confusion. Note also whether there is a smell of alcohol on the patient's breath. *Baseline observations should have been taken as soon as the patient arrived in the accident and emergency department, even before history and detailed examination.* This is most important.	
Systematic examination	RS	Think of the possibility of pneumothorax, haemothorax or lung damage
	CVS	Will give evidence of bleeding as stated above; there may also be signs such as atrial fibrillation and lung crackles, which suggest pre-existing heart disease

Reason for examination	Sign elicited	Comment
	CNS: Do the fullest neurological examination that the patient's level of consciousness permits	Statements such as 'neurological examination not possible because patient unconscious' must not be made
	Even in a patient who is totally unresponsive, neurological assessment is possible:	
	—are the respirations normal or are they laboured?	
	—does the patient gag when pharynx is aspirated?	Differences on the two sides of the body should be noted, as they may give the first sign of cerebral compression
	—if there are any spontaneous movements, are they symmetrical or is one side not moving as well?	
	—what are the reactions of the pupils?	
	—are the fundi normal or not?	
	—is there any evidence of papilloedema?	
	—are there retinal haemorrhages?	
	—is muscle tone normal?	
	—are the reflexes normal on both sides or not?	
	—what are the plantar reflexes?	

Injury to the head

Scalp lacerations, abrasions, haematomata, skin loss

It may be necessary to shave the head to exclude injury or to determine the nature of injury present

Any signs of fracture or depression of bone

Note the amount of bleeding that has occurred from the scalp

Much blood can be lost from scalp wounds

Bleeding from the nose

This may be due to fracture of the anterior cranial fossa or it may be due to damage to the nose

Bleeding from the ear

May be due to local injury, but often it is due to fracture of the petrous part of the temporal bone. Do not insert auriscope for fear of introducing infection and also damaging the ear drum

Get ENT opinion later

Leakage of cerebrospinal fluid from ear or nose (CSF otorrhoea or rhinorrhoea)

Test for glucose in the nasal fluid with a BM stick

If glucose present, the fluid is CSF and not due to a 'runny nose' ('it is not snot')

This is due to a tear in the meninges. The main danger is meningitis. Give sulphadiazine (a chemotherapeutic agent which crosses the blood–brain barrier well to give high concentrations in the CSF). Dose 1–1.5 g IM or IV every 4 hours for 2 days, followed by 1 g orally every 4 hours until leak stops. If renal impairment is present, high concentrations may cause toxic side effects such as nausea, vomiting, rashes, purpura and leucopenia

Reason for examination	Sign elicited	Comment
		If the patient with rhinorrhoea is conscious, he should be warned not to blow his nose because of the risk of increasing CSF leakage and also producing an intracranial aerocele
Injury to face, maxilla and mandible	Any facial deformity suggesting fractures? If the patient is conscious, can he open his mouth easily? If unconscious, can his mouth be opened? Examine mouth and remove dentures, blood or other foreign bodies which may still be present	The immediate danger from these fractures is respiratory obstruction. Tracheostomy may be necessary if the airway cannot be easily established or maintained. The help of an oral surgeon must be sought early in such cases
Injury to eyes	*The cornea:* there may be corneal abrasions or oedema which may show as diffuse haziness. The cornea may be lacerated	Corneal abrasions and haziness do not require specific treatment except eye toilet
	Conjunctiva: there may be conjunctival haemorrhage from rupture of a small conjunctival blood vessel	The posterior limit should be visible. The significance of such haemorrhage is that it may conceal injury to the deeper parts of the eye, and must be distinguished from sub-conjunctival haemorrhage (see below)

Anterior chamber: there may be bleeding in the anterior chamber; if slight, this will show as diffuse haziness of the aqueous humour and thus will make it difficult to visualize the details of the iris and fundus. In a few hours, the blood settles to the lowest part of the anterior chamber where it lies and shows as a fluid level. This is known as *hyphaema.* Sometimes the anterior chamber becomes filled with blood and this may lead to secondary glaucoma

The blood absorbs within a few days with rest

The iris: there may be dilatation of the pupil (mydriasis) due to damage to the third cranial nerve

The possibility of dilatation of the pupil due to cerebral compression must be borne in mind

There may be tears at the periphery of the iris

If small, they will heal spontaneously, but if large they will require repair

The lens: the lens may be dislocated after the injury

There will be defective vision after the injury.

Cataracts may occur shortly after the injury or many weeks later

If the patient complains of poor sight and this is not due to injury to the eyelids, he must be referred to an eye specialist urgently

More serious injuries include bleeding into the chamber, retinal detachment, rupture of the globe by blunt or penetrating injury, retention of foreign bodies

The main symptom is loss of vision. Such patients need urgent treatment. Eye injuries are a cause of much disability later, and need prompt and expert attention

275

Reason for examination	Sign elicited	Comment
		Other injuries include those to the orbit and optic canal
In injuries around the eye it is important to differentiate between a simple black eye and an orbital haematoma	An orbital haematoma is more likely if the following features are present: —changes confined to one side —the skin, though discolored, is intact —discoloration localized to the margin of the orbit and not extending outwards —external ocular movements may be impaired —subconjunctival haemorrhage (posterior limit not visible, unlike conjunctival haemorrhage where it is)	Simple black eye is due to direct injury, whereas orbital haematoma is due to fractures of the anterior and middle cranial fossae
Injury to chest	Check for damage to skin, for puncture wounds, flail segments, pneumothorax, haemothorax, fracture of ribs, injury to thoracic spine	These may give some evidence of the likelihood of damage to the heart or the great vessels Obtain a chest X-ray if in doubt
Injury to abdomen	Skin loss, bleeding wounds	
	Imprint of clothing on abdominal wall, puncture wounds penetrating into the abdominal cavity	If these features are present, it must be assumed, until proved otherwise usually by laparotomy, that damage has occurred to intra-abdominal viscera

	Tenderness, guarding, rigidity, and diminished bowel sounds	In the presence of a head injury, these signs cannot be relied on to indicate or disprove injury to an intra-abdominal viscus
	Palpable bladder	May be due to damaged urethra, to clot retention due to bleeding from the kidneys or bladder, or to urinary retention due to head injury
	Loin tenderness	This should alert you to the possibility of injury to the kidneys
Injury to the lumbar and sacral spines	Look for signs of injury to skin and subcutaneous tissue, for instance skin loss and haematoma Look for deformities which may indicate fracture of the spine	
Injury to the upper limbs and limb girdles	Fingers, wrists, forearms, arms, shoulders, scapulae, clavicles	Look for skin damage, bruising, deformity, pain, tenderness, and loss of function
Injury to lower limbs and limb girdles	Toes, feet, ankles, legs, knees, thighs, pelvis	In fractures of the pelvis, there is a risk of damage to intrapelvic organs, especially blood vessels with severe blood loss. Up to 2 litres of blood can be lost in fractures of the femur

277

Reason for examination	Sign elicited	Comment
Injury to the genitalia	Examine the genitalia especially in men Look for blood at the tip of the penis	This suggests damage to the urethra
	Palpate the shaft of the penis for any evidence of rupture of the urethra or to the rest of the organ	If there is any doubt about injury to the urethra, do not pass a urinary catheter: you will convert a partial rupture of the urethra into a complete one

What injuries are present? What investigations, if any, are required? Is the patient adequately resuscitated?

Urinalysis: Looking for blood. Indicated if there has been abdominal, loin or pelvic injury, and its presence suggests injury to the urinary tract.

Hb, group and save serum or cross match: Indicated where there has been blood loss or where there is a suspicion of blood loss. Also if an operation may be performed. In acute blood loss, haemoglobin is not a good measure of the amount of blood lost.

U&Es, glucose: Make sure head injury is not due to uraemia or hypo- or hyperglycaemia.

Skull X-rays: Much time is spent taking X-rays of the skull in patients with head injury. The student should appreciate the limitations of this investigation. On the one hand, the skull may not be fractured in severe trauma to the head. On the other, the skull is frequently fractured without significant damage to the brain. The following patients should be selected for skull X-ray:

1. Those who lost consciousness or cannot remember the head injury, or those whose Glasgow Coma Scale is 8 or less.
2. Those who have sustained a penetrating head injury, e.g. knife wound into the skull or gun shot wound.

3. Those in whom there are neurological symptoms (e.g. headaches, double vision) or signs (e.g. weakness, increased reflexes etc).
4. Those with CSF otorrhoea or rhinorrhoea.
5. Those who have bruising or swelling of the scalp.

X-ray of the neck: Must, in addition, be done in those who are unconscious or who may have had an injury to the neck. Ensure that you can see all cervical vertebrae. Other X-rays, for instance X-rays of the chest, abdomen, pelvis and limbs, should only be done in those in whom there is a suspicion of injury to these parts. They must not be done purely for medico-legal reasons. Also, in seriously injured patients, some of these X-rays can be delayed until the patient's condition has improved.

Blood alcohol level: This is valuable in those who smell of alcohol and who may have sustained a serious head injury. The alcohol level should be done early and repeated when it is considered that the effect of alcohol should have largely worn off. This gives an objective assessment of the patient's state of drunkenness, for, if the patient's level of consciousness remains depressed well after the level of alcohol has dropped, severe head injury is present.

Drug screening: Measure the levels of salicylate, barbiturates, paracetamol, phenytoin and other drugs if it is suspected that one of these agents has been accidentally or deliberately ingested.

Abdominal and chest X-rays: The value of abdominal and chest X-rays in patients who are suspected of bleeding internally must be appreciated. Significant bleeding within the thoracic cavity will lead to haemothorax which will show on a chest X-ray. If the chest X-ray is normal, then the chest cannot be the site of current bleeding. (The one exception to this is bleeding into the pericardial cavity. It takes only a small amount of blood in this cavity to produce fatal cardiac tamponade, and the X-ray features may not be helpful.) On the other hand, bleeding into the abdominal cavity cannot be diagnosed by X-ray.

Admit or discharge patient?

A patient who has had cerebral concussion and no

other injury, and has now fully recovered can be discharged home if the conditions below are met.

Concussion is a temporary state of unconsciousness produced by injury to the head. It produces paralysis which will often recover and does not result in structural damage to the brain. The patient will always have amnesia for the actual accident to the head. Death may occur because of inhalation of vomit or from failure of the respiratory centre to recover its function immediately. However, if the head injury was mild and no other injuries are present, the patient is fully conscious, and nervous system examination is normal, the patient can be discharged home. There should be a responsible adult to supervise the patient for the following 24 hours. The patient, and his relatives or friends who will look after him, must be given written information about those symptoms for which the patient must be brought back for further examination. These include persistent headaches, vomiting, neck pain and stiffness, photophobia, other visual disturbance such as double vision, weakness, convulsions and depression in conscious level.

The following patients should be admitted:

1. Those who are confused or have a depressed level of consciousness.
2. Those with neurological symptoms or signs.
3. Those with skull fractures.
4. Those who are difficult to assess because of alcohol, drugs, or medical conditions such as diabetes or epilepsy.
5. Those who do not have a responsible adult to supervise them, or those who have a social problem which makes management at home difficult.

Indications for referring patients with head injuries to neurosurgeons

1. Those with skull fractures with the following features:
   (a) Fracture depressed.
   (b) Patients with impaired levels of consciousness.
   (c) Patients with neurological symptoms (e.g. fits) or signs (e.g. muscle weakness).

2. Those with suspected base of skull fractures:
   (a) CSF otorrhoea or rhinorrhoea.
   (b) Bilateral orbital haematoma.
   (c) Penetrating injury.
3. Any patient who has the following features:
   (a) Impaired level of consciousness after resuscitation.
   (b) Deterioration in level of consciousness.
   (c) Any neurological impairment which has not subsided 8 hours after admission.

These patients will have CT scans of the brain on arrival. This investigation is now available in many hospitals that treat major trauma. If haematomas which are causing brain compression are found, they must be evacuated. Small haematomas are often observed and where necessary, CT scans repeated to show any change is size.

Case report

Features	Analysis
Mrs Elizabeth Spencer is a 45-year-old barmaid. She is married with two grown up sons. She was brought to the accident and emergency department by an ambulance following a road traffic accident 30 minutes earlier. The ambulance crew arrived 20 minutes after the accident and the journey to hospital took 10 minutes.	Note the patient's age and occupation. It is important to record the times of all major events relating to this accident. Times are measured in minutes, hours, days, etc. from the moment of the accident.
This patient had been well and free of all symptoms before this accident. She finished work in the pub where she worked as a barmaid and was given a lift home. She had drunk 3 glasses of white wine that evening. She was a passenger in the back seat of the car and was not wearing	Wherever possible, all relevant circumstances surrounding the accident should be recorded from the patient, eye witnesses, ambulance crew, etc. This lady had been drinking before this accident but do not let this distort your management of the patient. From the estimates of

Features	Analysis
a seat belt. The car she was in was going through traffic lights at about 25 miles an hour when it was hit by a car that went through red lights from the left side. The other car was estimated to be travelling at about 45 miles an hour.	the speeds and the amount of damage to the cars, this was a serious accident.
She was thrown sideways across her seat and the right side of her body hit the door. The impact was mainly to her head, shoulder and chest, but her neck was flung violently sideways. Her car was severely dented on the near (left) side and the other car had its front damaged.	She must be examined fully but pay particular attention to the right side of the body.
She did not remember the full details of the accident and claimed to have lost consciousness for 'a few minutes'. She remembered being freed from the damaged car, lying by the road side and later riding in the ambulance to hospital. According to the ambulance crew, she was deeply 'shocked' but was breathing normally. She gave her name correctly and told the crew that she had pain on the right side of her body. A cervical collar was applied before she was moved into the ambulance and her neck was handled gently.	There was a period of unconsciousness of uncertain duration but she seems to recall a number of events in this incident. Injured patients are often described as 'shocked' in the lay sense. Do not confuse this with clinical shock. Great care must be taken when handling an injured patient to protect the neck.

Rapid and preliminary examination in the A&E department showed she was not shocked and did not appear to require resuscitation. Glasgow Coma Scale was 15/15 and motor responses were symmetrical. Both pupils were normal and responded normally to direct and consensual illumination. BP was 110/60 and pulse 96/min and regular. Temperature was 36.8°C and respirations 18/min and of normal character.

As mentioned in the text, this is an important set of observations and must be taken and recorded accurately at the first opportunity. It could be done while the patient is being resuscitated. Important decisions about the patient's further management will depend on the progression of these observations.

On questioning, she denied having fits or double vision. She vomited partially digested food while waiting for the ambulance and complained that she had difficulty using her right upper limb due to pain in the arm.

Vomiting may be due to alcohol but may be due to brain injury. She may have injured her right arm but again, do not forget the possibility of motor deficit due to brain damage.

She also had a right sided pleuritic chest pain and mild difficulty breathing. She admitted to pain in her right calf, but she could move her lower limbs well.

Remember the right side of her body was the side of the impact. These sites may have been injured.

There were no other symptoms on systems enquiry. There was no significant past medical history and she was not taking any regular medications.

On examination she looked well though obviously distressed from the accident. She was not clinically shocked and had no pallor or cyanosis. There was a smell of alcohol on her breath.

Even though she does not need to be resuscitated, insert a good intravenous cannula now. This has been a serious injury and the patient will need IV fluids during the period of observation. Note again that the patient may be drunk, but do not let this cloud your judgement.

Features	Analysis
Heart sounds were normal and she was not in cardiac failure. She was tender over the right 4th to 8th ribs posteriorly. Percussion note was hyper-resonant and air entry diminished over the right side of her chest. There was no external sign of injury to the abdomen, which was soft and non-tender. The pelvis was normal. Bowel sounds were present and normal.	These are signs of a pneumothorax. It is encouraging that the abdomen and pelvis do not appear to have been seriously injured.
CNS examination showed no abnormalities apart from diminution of power in the right upper limb; this was thought to be due to injury to this arm.	Full CNS examination is mandatory in all patients with a head injury.
Systematic examination was carried out for injury. The following were found:	Make a note now of all injuries. They will need to be categorized in order of importance. This allows us to decide which treatments take precedence. The types of injury suspected or present dictate the kinds of investigations necessary.
—Large haematoma over the right parietal region of the scalp. There was no bleeding or leakage of CSF from the ears or the nose. There were no facial injuries.	
—The neck was tender on the right side on palpation.	
—She was tender over the right 4th to 8th ribs posteriorly. There were no puncture wounds or flail chest segments.	
—There was tenderness and a large haematoma around the mid portion of the right arm. All pulses in the limb were palpable and normal.	

Clinical diagnosis

1. Head injury with concussion. No evidence at the moment of serious brain injury or complications from trauma to the head. However, do not forget that there are indications, for instance the degree of damage to the vehicles, that this was a severe head injury. The extent of the injury beneath the right parietal haematoma is uncertain. A fracture of the skull cannot be excluded.
2. The soft tissues around the neck were injured. A fracture of the cervical spine cannot be ruled out.
3. Right pneumothorax, probably with fracture of one or more ribs from the 4th to 8th on the right.
4. The injury to the right arm is obviously to the soft tissues but the limitation of movement of the arm should raise the possibility of fracture of the humerus.

Investigations

Urinalysis was normal; there was no blood in the urine.

Hb was 13.3 g/dl.

Skull X-rays showed no fractures.

X-rays of the neck showed an intact cervical spine.

Chest X-ray showed a large right pneumothorax and fractures of the right 6th and 7th ribs. A small haemothorax was present at the base.

There was an undisplaced fracture of the mid shaft of the right humerus.

Negative urinalysis and skull X-ray do not of course exclude urinary tract and brain injury respectively.

A normal neck X-ray, however, is important, for it means the cervical spine is not fractured.

X-rays of the chest and the right humerus confirmed some of the injuries suspected.

Further observations and management

An intercostal tube drain was inserted on the right and the patient admitted for observation. The orthopaedic registrar was informed of the fracture of the humeral shaft and he applied a full arm sling and prescribed paracetamol for the pain.

Although injuries other than those to the head appeared to dominate the clinical picture, it was important to continue 'head injury' observations. The impact to the head appeared severe and there was loss of consciousness of uncertain duration.

Features	Analysis
The patient's blood pressure, pulse and respirations remained stable throughout but 6 hours after the accident, she started to complain of a headache and became restless. The Glasgow Coma Scale dropped to 9: she opened her eye only to pain (score 2); her best verbal response was inappropriate (3); and best motor response was withdrawal (4). It was noted that her left pupil was normal and responded to light shone in it. Her right pupil, on the other hand, was dilated and did not respond to light. However, light shone in the right eye made the left pupil contract.	Deterioration of the Glasgow Coma Scale and the pupillary signs are typical of acute intracranial bleeding. The bleeding could be into the extradural or subdural space. Note, also, that the side with the abnormal pupillary response is usually, but not necessarily, the side of the bleed. The signs may be due to indirect pressure on the third cranial nerve. The normal consensual light reaction of the left pupil means the optic nerve was intact.

Final diagnosis

CT scan confirmed a right subdural haematoma, which was successfully evacuated. Other diagnoses suggested by the history have been dealt with above.

Reference

Hope, R. A., Longmore, J. M., Hodgetts, T. J., Ramrakha, P. S. (1994) *Oxford Handbook of Clinical Medicine* (third edition). Oxford University Press, Oxford.

Index

287